From Broken to Blest:
Embracing the Healing That Awaits You

From Broken To Blest

Embracing the Healing That Awaits You

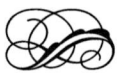

Adele M. Gill
with Dr. Verna Benner Carson

Silver Lining Communications, Inc.
www.silverliningcommunications.net

Unless otherwise noted, all Scripture quotations are from the New International Version Bible, (NIV), and the New American Bible (NAB) per online Bible Gateway.

From Broken to Blest:
Embracing the Healing That Awaits You
© Copyright 2017—Adele M. Gill with Dr. Verna Benner Carson

All rights reserved. Library of Congress copyright pending. No part of this publication may be reproduced, stored in a retrieval system or transmitted in any form or by any means—electronic, mechanical, photocopy, recording or any other—except for brief quotations in printed reviews, without the prior written permission of the publisher.

Registered to Silver Lining Communications Inc
ISBN: 978-0-578-19621-3 (print)
ISBN: 978-0-578-19622-0 (ebook)

This title is also available in e-book form.
Requests for information or for author contact, send email to:
silverliningcomm@gmail.com

Silver Lining Communications. Inc.
http://www.silverliningcommunications.net

Printed in the United States of America

Dedication

This book is dedicated to anyone who struggles with the effects of untreated childhood trauma, and subsequent, associated mind-body illness, especially depression, PTSD, autoimmune and/or neurological disorders in adulthood.

May they find life-changing healing through this book, and peace that surpasses understanding.

Acknowledgements

Special thanks to my family, Dr. Verna Benner-Carson, Harold Koenig, M.D., Efim Weinman, M.D., Karen Berg, LCSW, Adele Wilson, and Linda Vinciguerra for all their support and tireless efforts that have helped me to heal and bring this book, to press.

"Do not fear, for I am with you;

Do not be dismayed, for I am your God.

I will strengthen you and help you;

I will uphold you with my righteous right hand."

Isaiah 41:10 / Holy Bible (NIV)

Table of Contents

Foreword xiii
Introduction 1
Part I 7
  Chapter 1: Everyone Has a Past, Present, and a Future
  No One Is Exempt! 9
  Chapter 2: Birds of a Feather Really Do Flock Together 13
    The Good Fight 17
    Daddy & 'Uncle' Meyer at Saratoga Springs 19
    The Day That Changed Our Family Forever
    November 22, 1963 22
    Silver Lining 25
  Chapter 3: The 'At-Risk' Child 29
    The Unwelcome Visitor 33
    Mom's Homecoming 35
    The Butterfly 37
    Shasta & the 'Family Reunion' 38
    Homeless in the New York 44
    Silver Lining 47
  Chapter 4: Naming and Claiming Childhood Trauma 50
    The Captive Teen Years 51
    David and The 'Age of Freedom' 56
    Howie's Big Exit 58
    Howie, Charlie and the First "Apalachin" Meeting 61
    Choosing to Live in Today 65
    Remembering Childhood Trauma 69
    Silver Lining 75

Chapter 5: Uncharted Waters: The College Years 78
   Living on the Edge 78
   The Reef 82
   A New Beginning 87
   St. Joseph's Hospital School of Nursing 89
   Silver Lining The Serenity Prayer 91
Chapter 6: Settling Down 93
   The Love of My Life 93
   Realizing My Dream 95
   Here I Am! 97
   The Unpaved Road 104
   Leaving Work on Disability 106
   Silver Lining 109
Chapter 7: Untreated Childhood Trauma 111
   Untreated Childhood Trauma &
   the Depression Epidemic 114
   Dr. Scott and the Medical Merry-Go-Round 122
   Our Big Blessing 126
   Accepting My Own Mind-Body Disconnect 128
   Silver Lining 136
Chapter 8: The Mind-Body-Faith Phenomenon 138
   Inpatient Hospitalization: On the Brink of Despair 138
   No Blame, No Shame 144
   New Life: The Joy of the Lord is my Strength 149
    Wheelchair Time 151
   Another Chance 154
   Confusion in the ER 158
   Silver Lining 161
Chapter 9: Silent No More, Victim No More 167
   Silver Lining 176
   Silver Lining 183

Chapter 10: Moving From Broken to Blest 184
    7 Steps to Move From Broken to Blest 184
    Step 1 Acknowledge Your Brokenness 185
    Step 2: Ask Jesus to Come Into Your Life 186
    Step 3: Put Aside All Worry and Fear 189
    Step 4: Reach For Forgiveness 191
    Step 5: Accepting Your Own Imperfections & Those of Others 195
    Step 6: Learn to Look For Silver Linings in Adversity ... 196
    Step 7: Embrace the Healing That Awaits You 199
    Silver Lining 200
Chapter 11: Time to Banish Negative Thinking 202
Chapter 12: Contentment: I Have All That I Need 206
    The Secret of Contentment 206
    Silver Lining 209
Chapter 13: ~ Gratitude, Peace & Joy 211

Epilogue 217
Part II: The Healing Workshop 219
    Chapter 1 Questions 221
    Chapter 2 Questions 228
    Chapter 3 Questions 235
    Chapter 4 Questions 243
    Chapter 5 Questions 250
    Chapter 6 Questions 255
    Chapter 7 Questions 262
    Chapter 8 Questions 269
    Chapter 9 Questions 276
    Chapter 10 Questions 282
    Chapter 11 Questions 289
    Chapter 12 Questions 293
    Chapter 13 Questions 297

Healing Workshop Questions	305
Workshop Questions: Moving From Broken to Blest	309
Memory Lane: A Place to Visit, Not to Dwell	317
The Healing Journal Workshop	321
References	331
Resource Books	333
Prayers	335

Foreword

By Harold G. Koenig, M.D.

When I was asked to write the foreword to this book, I felt quite honored. At the time of the request I did not personally know Adele M. Gill. However, Adele's co-author, Dr. Verna Benner Carson is not only a good friend of mine but a collaborator with me on many publications and public presentations. I knew that if Verna was involved, that the manuscript had to be excellent and indeed it is.

From Broken to Blest: Embracing the Healing That Awaits You is a compelling, riveting story, a powerful case study/memoir of one woman's journey living with brokenness due to untreated childhood trauma, and later, subsequent mind-body illness throughout adulthood.

Reading this extraordinary book could be life-changing, even life-saving, for anyone who has felt unloved or not good enough in their life as a result of untreated childhood trauma or other trauma.

Adele grew up with a mother who was mentally ill and was hospitalized in a mental institution for a year and a half when she was just 6 years old. Her father was in the Mafia and began introducing Adele to his 'underworld life' around the age of 4. As a result of being the focus of her mother's harsh angst, and witnessing her father's underworld activities first-hand, she endured significant, untreated childhood trauma throughout her youth. Adele went on to experience severe mind-body effects throughout her adult life, due to the untreated childhood trauma she endured in her youth.

Brokenness experienced in childhood often leaves people

unable to make sense out of their pain later in life. Adele's journey is a testament to the ability of God to heal and restore mind-body wholeness, even in the face of adversity. Her story exemplifies challenges associated with Health and Spirituality, a far-reaching topic I have written about for decades together with my colleague, Dr. Verna Benner Carson, the co-author of this book. Adele's story is one of untreated childhood trauma, and subsequent disability and infirmity, endurance, resilience, forgiveness, healing, redemption, and eventually, by the grace of God, triumph. Most of all, it is a bold witness to the healing power of prayer and placing one's trust in the hands of a loving, merciful, faithful God.

In 2010, while struggling with the daily challenges of her mind-body illness, Adele discovered a concept that she calls the *Mind-Body-Faith Phenomenon©*. She has continued to explore and develop this theory together with the co-author of this book, Dr. Verna Benner Carson. As a result of the *Mind-Body-Faith Phenomenon©*, which includes prayer and belief in God's healing power, Adele has been able to heal, experience maximal wellness, and has abundant peace and joy to share with others.

In addition to Adele's compelling story, this book also offers readers the extraordinary opportunity to go *from broken to blest* in their own lives through *The Healing Workshop* section of the book. *The Healing Workshop* was developed with the understanding that some readers may experience a stirring of their own painful childhood trauma issues through reading this book. That is, after reading this book, some may experience the pain associated with memories long forgotten, denied and put aside. The co-authors of *From Broken to Blest:*

Embracing the Healing That Awaits You have developed and shared this valuable resource section, *The Healing Workshop*, to gently help readers who have experienced emotional trauma to heal in body, mind and spirit. *The Healing Workshop* provides readers with the opportunity to gently revisit those memories in a healing context. In that way, for people who are open to their own truth, this book may truly be a God send.

From Broken to Blest: Embracing the Healing That Awaits You

> *"Finally, brothers and sisters, whatever is true,
> whatever is noble, whatever is right, whatever is pure,
> whatever is lovely, whatever is admirable–if anything is excellent or
> praiseworthy–think about such things."*
>
> Philippians 4:8

1. Identify Negative Thoughts As They Occur
2. Banish Negative Thoughts
3. Escort Negative Thoughts Out Promptly
4. Focus on Positive Imagery (such as a favorite place)
5. Surround Yourself With Positive People
6. Stay Busy
7. 'Speak Life' into every circumstance and relationship

Introduction

The fact that you are reading this book, *From Broken to Blest: Embracing the Healing That Awaits You*, tells me you or a loved one may very well be weary, know brokenness first-hand, and be in need of healing.

Whatever it is that led you to read this book, perhaps it is "meant to be" that you have this particular book in your hands right now. *From Broken to Blest: Embracing the Healing That Awaits You* is my own personal true-life story—one of unrelenting, ongoing, untreated childhood trauma, and subsequent depression, PTSD, and 35 years of living with subsequent, associated autoimmune and neurological illness.

Most of all, my story, my witness is about the power of forgiveness, redemption, and ultimately wholeness in the arms of Jesus. Though it has taken some five decades for me to discern and gather the courage to share my own life story, doing so has brought me tremendous healing in mind, body and soul. For me, this healing journey has been more like climbing a massive, steep mountain, or removing shrapnel, than simply peeling off the proverbial onion layers.

After initially seeing 70 medical doctors with various specialties and many acute care hospitalizations, I was still virtually undiagnosed and finally realized that this was not my own battle to fight. Clearly, this was a 'God job' if there ever was one!

As a direct result of the childhood trauma that I endured, I emerged from my youth into adulthood with life-threatening physical disabilities from damage sustained to both my immune and neurological systems from childhood trauma. With depression, and post-traumatic stress disorder, also known as PTSD, I also need to use a bipap respirator 12-14 hours per 24 hour day for mechanical respiratory support. I live with frequent exacerbations of difficulty breathing, garbled speech, difficulty swallowing when fatigued, respiratory and generalized muscle weakness due to an unspecified progressive neuromuscular condition the doctors call myasthenia-like syndrome.

In my life, writing my own story has been key to healing—emotionally, medically and spiritually. Necessary--to begin the restorative process in mind, body and spirit.

Before writing my story, I found it difficult to put my childhood trauma experiences into words and it was very hard to share them with others in a way they could understand. The intensity and pain of my childhood was hard for me to accept as, in a sense, it was unspeakable, due to the extent of what I endured. What is written here is just a small part of what transpired in my youth, particularly with my father and his 'activities.' There is so much more I could have written but chose not to, as it is just too painful.

Over the past 10 years, because of my mind-body health, and being flooded with childhood flashbacks and nightmares, I have been forced to come to terms with the memories of my youth and my parents and grow in forgiveness by being able to pray for them both. That has been a big challenge for me as my mother suffered dearly from what I have been told was ultimately major depression and untreated paranoid schizophrenia. My father was a marginal character always seeming to be running from the law, who, in my considered opinion, did not seem to know right from wrong or have a conscience. In that way, because of this, Dad was a very good fit for the double life he led in the Mob, with Meyer Lansky, his mentor, and his other seasonedunderworld 'associates.'

Not sure why, but my writing this book has been met with some family resistance. When asked, my siblings have only shared brief experiences and memories of our childhood without 'connecting the dots' so to speak, as I was forced to do because of my health issues. Though I'm sure we were all affected by our childhoods, they are both fortunately, in good health living full lives. I can only conclude that based on how we grew up, we are all just doing the best we can to deal with the memories and perspectives we each have. It is as if each of us was raised by different parents. My relationship with my siblings is very important to me, as they are precious people in my life—always have been, and always will be. The fact is that much happened in my young life when they were not there. I'm not sure why my father singled me out and chose to intimately include me in his underworld, especially from middle school on, after my sister went away to college. But he did. In a capsule, my siblings did not witness the full extent of Dad's 'activities' as he revealed to me the sordid side of his double life. Due to work and college, my siblings were not there as the years pressed on with Dad's weekend 'activities' with me in tow.

Though they were aware, they were not the focus of my mother's abusive cruelty, hostility, angst, and raging anger that she directed toward me increasingly in my teenage years.

Yes, I was a victim in my youth, but today I am 'silent no more and victim no more' as I share here how the love of God has saved me from an unspeakable life of early trauma, brokenness and feeling unloved. In actuality, I now see myself as a servant of God, and a witness to His holy love in my life, and am fully committed to sharing my witness.

From Broken to Blest is my personal story, my own witness of what I have seen God do in my life since my traumatic youth. I am free to share with others about my tumultuous, traumatic childhood, even in print for the first time, but most of all, I am free to tell others about how God saved me from childhood trauma and a life of torment. Free at last!

Perhaps my father saw me as someone who could unwittingly assist him in building his organization as I was so outgoing and precocious in my youth. These qualities helped him meet people easily, many whose family members later became "business associates" in what Dad often referred to as, 'The Syndicate,' 'The Racket,' 'Our Thing,' 'The Outfit,' 'Cosa Nostra,' and 'Meyer's American Mafia.' In a way, it seems that my father used me as an unwitting shield, a decoy, a favorite fishing lure to grow his organization.

Today, by any measure, I still face seemingly insurmountable mind-body health challenges, yet that is just a small part of my story. In actuality, my story is a witness to how God, through Hisunmatched, unconditional love, grace, mercy, and forgiveness, has raised me up on eagles' wings from the depths of untreated childhood trauma, subsequent despair and adulthood infirmity.

Despite it all, God has brought me abundant peace, joy, healing in body, mind, and spirit, and new life to share with others, in Jesus Christ, and for that I am eternally grateful.

By the grace of God, through writing this book over the past 6 years, I have experienced significant physical and emotional healing. Writing my story has provided me with tremendous catharsis and has helped me deal with lifelong depression and anxiety, gain confidence, and build self-esteem that was trampled in my traumatic youth. Most of all, sharing my witness has offered me the great privilege to recognize and share with others how Jesus has interceded on my behalf again and again, to protect, comfort and guide me through uncharted, turbulent waters.

It is not uncommon for traumatic childhood memories to take root and cause serious damage, involving both physical and mental health later in adult life, particularly neurological and/or autoimmune conditions. That is exactly what happened in my life. For me, frank and open self-acceptance, with a 'no shame, no blame' philosophy, and ongoing therapy, has provided me with a strong sense of relief, and a much better understanding of who I am and what I have endured in my youth. By so doing, I have effectively been able to lay down my childhood burdens for the first time ever after repressing the early trauma for five decades, affecting my overall health and wellness. I am now far more able to recognize, and share life with others the blessings, compassion and grace that God has seeded in my. It is with a full and grateful heart that I am able to press on and move forward, striving to live life to the fullest each day with peace and joy.

By the grace of God, for the glory of God, after five decades of silence, I am now able to remember, talk about, and write about what happened in my youth, to connect the dots, so to speak, to grieve innocence lost, and through prayer, to grow in forgiveness for those who hurt me most. I will never be able to thank God enough for preserving me through those traumatic years and throughout my adulthood. It is my express hope that by sharing my story here, it will benefit others who are trapped in the muck and mire, the quicksand, of untreated childhood trauma, and the associated negative, hopeless feelings and infirmity that often accompanies it. Moreover, it is my expressed hope and prayer that they will also find Jesus in the process, and through Him, be able to heal and live full and productive lives.

The signature Bible verse for *From Broken to Blest: Embracing the Healing That Awaits You* is from Acts 26:16-18 [NIV]:

"I have appeared to you to appoint you as a servant and as a witness of what you have seen and will see of me. I will rescue you from your own people..."

This Scripture reveals the purpose for writing this book about my traumatic childhood, and about the Almighty, loving, healing hand of God that has comforted and protected me in my youth and throughout adulthood.

Through this book, this witness, I hope I can help others who have suffered from untreated childhood trauma to protect, improve, and restore their own physical and mental health.

From Broken to Blest: Embracing the Healing That Awaits You is written not only for trauma survivors, but also for, parents, teachers, social workers, nurses, doctors and clergy---in fact for anyone who is in a position to make a significant, life-saving and life-giving difference in the life of anyone of any age who is enduring, or has endured, childhood or other emotional trauma.

*Due to the sensitive nature of this witness, some names and locations have been changed to protect anonymity.

Part I

CHAPTER 1:
Everyone Has a Past, Present, and a Future
No One Is Exempt!

"I have appeared to you to appoint you as a servant and as a witness of what you have seen and will see of Me."

Acts 26:16

Everyone has a childhood story, and here, in this book, is where I have chosen to share my story, my witness. What I have lived, and subsequently, what I have seen of the Lord in my own life, in my 60 years of living. It is my express hope that by telling my story, others will be encouraged to seek God in earnest, accept Jesus into their lives, and to heal from trauma in their own lives.

In this book, as in the above Scripture says, I give witness not only to my turbulent early life and living with untreated childhood trauma, but especially to God, who is my strength, my shield, my refuge and my saving grace.

I think it is fair to say I did not grow up in a *'Leave it to Beaver'* type family. I grew up in Utica, a small town in Upstate New

York, and then later in the DC area with my two siblings, with an abusive mother who suffered dearly, it seems, with untreated major depression and schizophrenia, and struggled with paranoia, agitation, and was psychotic most of the time. With little if any support, my mother suffered in every way, and as a result, so did we.

Due to her mental illness, Mom struggled mentally, emotionally, physically, financially, socially, and spiritually to function independently while trying to raise 3 children on her own. My father left when I was about 10 years old to live across town with his 'other family' and though I did not know it then, to pursue his double life with Meyer Lansky and the Mob. I can only imagine how hard it all must have been for my mother!

Clearly, to all who knew them, there were great disparities between my parents' worlds and approaches to everything regarding parenting, morality, pro-life issues and values, politics, religion -- atheism vs orthodox Roman Catholicism, Dad's Mob 'activities,' and life in general, was epic. I simply cannot fathom how they ever could have gotten along well enough to marry.

In a way, it's hard for me to even imagine how my parents ever married as their perspectives on religion, politics, child rearing and the world-at-large and – and, indeed all things that matter most— were so disparate.

In our family, it is as if all 3 of us were raised by different parents. Siblings often, for various reasons, often have very different experiences growing up in the same family, as every parent-child relationship is dynamic and unique. Additionally, each child may process what occurred in her/his youth differently, as is the case in my family.

Some deal with childhood trauma through denial of what was, yet others carefully and purposefully wrap their traumatic experience within a cloak of loyalty and silence, both of which characterize my family to some degree. In my case, finally telling my story is very freeing. By so doing, I am shedding the 'don't tell' family mantra and the all-inclusive shroud of secrecy that prevailed in my family. However, now I am 'silent no more.' Having lived with mental illness in my family, mental and physical abuse, poverty and neglect, as well, my own issues, I find my life story is a pressing one that must be told; a story that must be shared because of my final conclusion: Jesus is the greatest hope I have ever known, especially in the face of the unrelenting day in day out childhood trauma I experienced and its mind-body connection fall-out in adulthood.

It is, indeed ironic that my mother was the one who intentionally instilled in me strong faith.

During her infrequent lucid times, she talked incessantly about 'being Catholic.' She had great devotion to Blessed Mother Mary, Jesus and the Holy Spirit, and had a beautiful picture of Mary and baby Jesus at the end of her bed. During her psychotic rants, I would quietly gaze at Blessed Mother's picture and pray God would give me a gentle, kind mother like Mary. Though that did not happen in my youth, I learned to grow in compassion for my own mother's plight as I got older, and came to understand the extent of her mental illness and health challenges, in part because I have had my own struggles with depression and infirmity.

The difference was that I have had a strong support system in my adult life. Even in the toughest times, at a very early age, by my calculations around 6 years of age, I learned to trust in Jesus, and for that, I have never been disappointed, and am eternally grateful for the life and the witness God has provided me. For in this life, we all experience the blessed, the good, the bad, and the ugly. Since my childhood, I have experienced some difficult life experiences, trials, fear and anxiety, sadness, disappointments, rejection, abandonment, and hurts that could have obscured my path, and affected my world-view, even making me bitter, as is often the case of victims of childhood trauma. But by the grace of God, it did not! Instead, these experiences helped me grow in faith as I was eventually able to go from broken to blest with God's help.

Whatever you have endured, your reactions depend on your ability to choose to reframe memories and to embrace a healthy perspective. This is a choice I have made for myself, to process life experiences in a positive way as they evolve. Though my own childhood was quite unusual and traumatic, I have chosen to look at my childhood through the eyes of faith. And my conclusion is, that God chose the family of my birth specifically for me, long before I was even conceived. In His infinite wisdom, I was exactly where I was meant to be in my youth, and it prepared me for my later adult life in the most blessed ways. Ironically, some of the same skills I developed as a child living in my chaotic family of origin, now help me cope with daily living with a progressive degenerative neuromuscular condition.

CHAPTER 2:
Birds of a Feather Really Do Flock Together

"I can do all things through Christ Who gives me strength."

Philippians 4:11-13 / NIV

My father, Howie, was a Bronx-born 'Good Fella,' who spent a lot of time in my youth with his 'business associates' including Meyer Lansky, his mentor. I learned from spending time with Dad and his 'associates' at an very early age, that *'Birds of a feather really do flock together.'*

Born in 1924, of German ancestry, my father, Howie, saw a lot growing up and seemed to revel in his early Bronx roots— where he spent a lot of time on the streets and docks of New York City. Well-educated, a mechanical engineer by trade, he served in the Navy, and went to Stevens Institute of Engineering, Hoboken, New Jersey.

Though we kids were all too young to really understand the full gravity and origin of his frequent Bronx-based 'bedtime stories,' on occasion, Dad would discretely tell us three kids his covert versions of some of the action-packed antics of some of the unusual, tough, underworld characters and legends he knew from his youth and beyond. And all this after my Mom would sing us Ave Maria at bedtime then leave the room.

As a young child, I used to marvel at the characters in Dad's occasional bedtime stories. In fact, I preferred his bedtime stories to him reading books as he and my mother often did in the early years growing up. Of course he was always careful not to divulge his connections to the characters in his stories. Little did I know until some four decades later, that some of his bedtime stories were at least in part, based in truth. I'm sure some of the characters were from his youth in the Bronx and then New Jersey where he went to college in Hoboken and where he later held meetings with his Jersey cousin, John.

It is noteworthy that my childhood memories of Howie's world were blocked for decades. It was as if I had just enough puzzle pieces to get a rough outline of his underworld life, just the gist, but not a full picture. However, by the grace of God, over a span of many years into adulthood, I slowly received one puzzle piece at a time through memories, flashbacks and nightmares. Through many 'aha' moments, I eventually was able to understand the 'finer nuances' of his sordid double life. Looking back, I suspect God knew it was too much for me to embrace all at once in my youth so the Lord shielded me until I was much older, was in therapy, and more prepared for the gravity of what I learned about his life.

Dad had many friends and associates in our neighborhoods where we lived while I was growing up in Upstate New York—and even in Takoma Park, Maryland where we later moved with Mom after they divorced. Several of Howie's neighbor friends in Upstate New York reportedly were in jail for many years, while their wives worked hard to keep things going at home for and with their young children. Some were our neighbors and friends. In fact, we had three neighbors whose fathers were all Dad's friends, and all reportedly in jail at the same time, for what I do not know.

After leaving engineering in the late 60' where he worked as a mechanical engineer with aerospace and electronics, Dad generally did not discuss his 'new' occupation with us kids even when we were older. As the years passed by, his lack of communication ultimately allowed each of us to draw our own conclusions as to what he really did.

Sometimes he said he worked selling corrugated boxes with a company in New Hampshire.

Though my siblings seemed to take him at his word, I always found it hard to believe that he went from being a bright mechanical engineer to selling corrugated boxes. For more than a few years I thought he was in the CIA, However, as the years pressed on, he left a long crumb trail of clues as to his 'double life' as a 'Good Fella.'

It is noteworthy that of the three of us, I am the only one who has pursued, recognized and accepted that Howie led a double life. Though my siblings were also there with me on many occasions early on, they too seem to have memory blocks on details similar to those I used to have, including places and names of people we met, and they seemed to have no overt desire to remember these things. As the years pressed on, they were not there for many of his adventures as they were working and away at college, but he still came and picked me up and took me with him to meetings.

Howie would conjure up fun activities and plans to keep of us busy while he held his Mob meetings with his associates. We hiked, swam, climbed rocks at the King and Queens' seat in Maryland, hiked at state parks, went 'diamond hunting' for quartz while climbing on tall cliffs in Herkimer, NY, swimming at lakes in the Adirondacks, and spelunking deep in dark caves without any equipment whatsoever. I was not outdoorsy at all, and had little interest in leaving his side, but my brother and sister loved his fun adventures, and these activities served as a distraction for them from his meetings as they went off to do the activity of the day with me choosing to stay behind at Dad's side.

After my sister, who is three years older than me, went away to college in 1971 when I was about 14 years old, my brother got a part time weekend job as a janitor's helper at the local Catholic church. On weekends, Dad would drive from Middle River, Maryland where he lived to Takoma Park, Maryland, pick me up and drive an hour and a half to his 'recruitment headquarters.' By

1985, I also had the added 'benefit' of knowing many people who knew Howie after my husband and I unwittingly moved close to the area where Howie met with most of his contacts in the 70's.

To this day, I still pray fervently and often for Howie and those who fell prey to his charming demeanor, as he carefully, informally, profiled everyone he met to meet his subversive criteria for possible inclusion in his activities' and 'organization,' either as a compadre, a partner, or an unwitting victim. Over the years I have realized that he especially looked for trusting, vulnerable people with large families, especially those with drinking fathers and distracted, devout, Catholic, church going mothers, some with ADHD, some with rebellious, drug or alcohol addicted children who were vulnerable. In many cases, in most of the communities we went to, he had a series of girlfriends that he 'lived' with—just part of his M.O.

As a young girl, from middle school on, I often asked Dad about his job, and he would flatly respond to my inquiries by saying, *"What do you think I do?"* and then, change the subject or continue reading the stock pages in the local newspaper. Dad was a complex man—a rather charming, eccentric character who had many diverse interests and 'activities,' who was always also very much of a calculating, unconventional man, and a utilitarian opportunist, seemingly anti-Christian, and certainly anti-Catholic. Though to me Howie seemed to be devoid of a conscience, he was a fearless, curious, unusual, adventurous and interesting mystery man to me and most who knew him, one that people seemed to follow blindly.

Mom, on the other hand, was an overly scrupulous soul—a proud, feisty Bostonian, and an orthodox Roman Catholic who thought that Pope John Paul II was 'not Catholic enough.' She made us genuflect on the sidewalk when we would pass the Catholic Church on the hard concrete. She hated it when the Mass was no longer celebrated in Latin, and cherished every stringent dogma the Catholic Church had to offer. In fact, if she felt there weren't adequate Catholic rules in place for things, she actually often made them up. One of Mom's made up rules was that if we were late for Mass on Sunday we needed to attend two masses to "make up" for being late. The fact that we had no means of transportation and had to walk two miles just to get to church had no bearing with Mom at all – we were late and that was a sin. Having to attend two masses each Sunday because we were always late due to no transportation to church and walking about two miles to get there each way was enough to make anyone hate church!

Mom was a very strict disciplinarian, a stay at home mom, then later a secretary for the federal government, but always had wanted to be a Catholic nun. She was extremely rigid, a woman who had scrupulous integrity, which made it hard for anyone to relate to her, including and especially family, as her idea of right and wrong was solidly black and white, with no room for shades of gray. Mom also lived with severe depression and OCD, or Obsessive Compulsive Disorder. Her hand washing, repetitive behaviors turning on and off stove flames and house lights only became more pronounced and disruptive to her life—and ours--with each passing year. It was as if she had seen something that haunted her, and the only way she knew to deal with it was through repetition and trying to wash her hands again and again to ease the pain of her lingering memories.

THE GOOD FIGHT

One day, when my mother was 6 months pregnant with me, around March 1957, she was sitting in the front row of church at Mass, and had a grand mal seizure. It was the first seizure she had ever experienced. Subsequently, she was diagnosed with epilepsy while pregnant with me and placed on dilantin and phenobarbital. When my mother went home from church and told my Dad about what happened, my mother said Dad was reportedly worried that something must be wrong with the baby she was carrying (me), and pressured her hard to abort me. Being a devout Roman Catholic, she adamantly refused, even as he insisted in every way to abort me.

From that time on, Mom later told me that her marriage was never the same; that Dad no longer wanted her, or me either, for that matter. In light of all this, and the stigma associated with having epilepsy, it was nothing short of a miracle when my mother and Howie went on to have a third child, my brother, just 16 months after I was born. I must have been in middle school, perhaps around 14 years old, when my mother first told me, for the first time, in a psychotic rage about Howie wanting her to abort me. Apparently, he was sure something was wrong with me. I was absolutely crushed. The thought that Dad did not want her, or me, was absolutely overwhelming to me for many years, and I quietly began to sink into depression in my adolescence.

At first, I felt deeply hurt by what she told me when she was in this psychotic fit of rage.

However, many years later, I realized one day that actually meant she must have fought with everything she had for me to be born...what a blessing! This reframed realization turned my thoughts and feelings from deep rejection and shame to deep gratitude for my mother's determination and fortitude to preserve my life.

The thought that Mom fought hard for me and was unbending with Dad in whether or not I should be born eventually became pure joy for me much later in adulthood. You see, though my relationship with Mom was turbulent and difficult due to her acute, untreated mental illness, I came to see the struggle she must have had on my behalf with Howie pressing her to abort me.

In a way, she laid down her life and marriage for her Catholic faith – and for me— I will always be eternally grateful!

Fast Forward

Mom and I attended the first March on Washington together to protest Rowe vs Wade together with Catholic church and thousands of other protesters. This event went on to become an Annual Pro-life March, and was one of the best memories we ever shared as we were completely joined in purpose that day. She even let me skip school to attend, which was a first. We rode a chartered bus together to the area near the reflecting pools and sang songs and held picket signs with throngs of parishioners from all across the US protesting abortion. It was the best day Mom and I had together ever!

Daddy & 'Uncle' Meyer at Saratoga Springs

In the early 60's, when I was about 5 years old, my family went camping at Pesico Lake near Saratoga Springs in Upstate New York. We set up camp, then, Dad announced he and I were going to look around town to get the lay of the land. That was the first time I had ever met his associate, 'Uncle Meyer.' I was told to call him 'Uncle' Meyer- I never did know his last name until I was in my forties. When we returned back to our campsite many hours later, it was almost dark and my father had been drinking heavily, which was not uncommon.

Brimming with excitement he told Mom he had an 'important impromptu meeting' with a man named Meyer at the nearby Saratoga Raceway in Saratoga Springs, New York, *"Howie, how could you do this to me?"* Mom asked. In his usual logical, charming way, he was able to convince her it was simply a coincidence that his friends were there, and that he never meant to stay so long, but that they had to meet about something very important.

The next day, Howie found another reason to leave the campsite to return and go back to the Saratoga Springs Racetrack. This time he took both my older sister and me with him, saying my brother was too young to go and had to stay back at the campground with Mom. When Dad and 'Uncle' Meyer were finished talking about the new Saratoga racetrack, the unions, casinos, gambling, trafficking, and money, it was time to return to the campground. Again, like the day before, when he had returned from the racetrack, Dad had been drinking. He drove us back to our campsite where Mom sat fuming as my little brother had fallen asleep in her arms. My parents argued loudly into the night about his spending so much time with his friends and associates. She had good reason to be annoyed with Howie's compadres. Reportedly, his closest friend and associate 'Cody,' actually even had showed up in Niagara Falls, New York on their honeymoon to meet with Howie!

When I woke up in the morning, there was still a good bit of tension in the air, and Mom and Dad were taking down the little awning attached to the camper, as Mom announced that vacation was over, and we were going home. From looking at my Mom's expression, I knew it was true.

We were going home after just a day and a half, despite the fact that our vacation had barely started. But it had been lots of fun anyway—despite Dad leaving Mom to be with 'Uncle' Meyer.

Fast Forward

Some four decades later, when I was in my 40's after first being introduced to 'Uncle' Meyer at Saratoga Racetrack in Saratoga Springs, New York, I was on my bipap respirator one afternoon watching TV, and I noticed a very familiar face in the corner of my eye on the TV screen. It was 'Uncle' Meyer! The man Howie had often called by the nickname 'Luigi,' but I knew him as 'Uncle Meyer,' was on TV! To my great surprise, and my utter dismay, it was a History Channel documentary called, "The New York Mafia: The Five Families of New York" and it featured none other than my Howie's close mentor, 'Uncle Meyer,'–who apparently also was known as an infamous New York mobster, and some of Dad's other associates!

Though I had often heard about Meyer Lansky while was meeting with other Mob associates, and seen 'Uncle' Meyer many times with Howie when I was really young, I had never connected the dots before, never asked his last name. At that time, all I knew was that the man on the TV was my dad's longtime mentor whom I had been told to call, 'Uncle Meyer' as a young girl, some 45 years earlier. Though the clues were all there, I was shocked at his association with the Mob, as Howie had used every other word to describe his world besides the term, 'Mafia,' like the Syndicate, Our Thing, The Racket, The Entertainment Industry, and the Unions. Yet, deep in my heart, as I got older, I knew that the Mob was Howie's world. Feeling like I needed to know more about his associates and Howie's world, I went to the local Barnes & Noble book store, found the crime section and then the 'Mafia Encyclopedia' to read more about Meyer Lansky. How could this possibly be??? Aghast at what I saw, I will never forget that day as I sat dumb-founded, heart racing while pouring over the book photos and stories of many of Howie's close associates whom I had met, including 'Uncle' Meyer. I recognized many of the men by their faces, nicknames and localities. Howie had always been extremely careful not to reveal real names and locations whenever he took me with him to meet his associates. Last names were always covert or omitted, and many went by nicknames like Luigi ('Uncle' Meyer Lansky).

I remember being in shock and speechless, as I learned about Howie's world that day, and who his New York and New Jersey 'associates' really were. In fact, I later learned that my life with Dad seemed to follow important Mob events. Many pictures in the book were familiar faces, and included places Dad had taken me with him to New York and New Jersey so many times where he met with his compadres when I was really young.

When I was very young, it was not uncommon for Dad to start loud arguments with my mother on Fridays, where he would come pick me up and take me with him telling her he would be away for the weekend. Looking back, I think it was actually a predictable ploy that allowed him to leave the house for 3 days at a time-with a reason. Often, he would take me with him, and go to New Jersey and New York City and drop me off in the care of strangers ~ his Italian descent associates and their families. Who would suspect anyone of any wrong doing from someone with a young child in tow as a shield, decoy, a distraction?

As a result of growing up in our severely dysfunctional family, my parents had everything to do with my growing in empathy for others. Likewise, they are responsible for the person I am today, as my greatest desires is to love my family, serve the poor and homeless, and to trust in the Triune God.

Mom tried hard to live her Catholic faith to the letter, and she taught me everything I needed to know about faith by the time I was 6 years old. Paradoxically, though my mother was the orthodox Catholic one in our family who led me to Blessed Mother Mary, Jesus, and the Holy Spirit, it was my father, Howie, who was the one who especially led me to God himself. This happened as my youth pressed on, when I eventually realized my earthly father was not to be emulated nor trusted, and was incapable of love. I loved him, but hated the fact it did not seem to be reciprocal. Putting aside all loyalty he instilled in me, I eventually realized, to my dismay, that he was the polar opposite of Father God in every way! It is my belief that Mom's fervent prayers, through the power of the Holy Spirit, saved me from much heartache and danger in my youth, and I carry that with me always.

Adele M. Gill

The Day That Changed Our Family Forever November 22, 1963

Walking into the room, I saw Gammy, my grandmother, and my mother, talking seriously, in hushed tones about something seemingly important. Gammy often came to visit when things got really hard to deal with at our house. She was keenly aware of the dynamic my parents had, and was most generous in every way in helping our family deal with Mom's mental illness as she came to visit about every 6 months.

As I entered the room, I remember asking what happened.

"The president has been shot" Mom said as she dried her tears with a tissue. *"He was Catholic, and he was from Boston where my family came from. He was a wonderful president, but someone killed him. He was a good man and we are sorry to see him go.*

"Who could have done such a thing?" I asked.

"Not everyone likes the Kennedys" my grandmother interjected with deep certainty, as she, too, stoically wiped her tears away. *"Why,"* I persisted, *"didn't everyone like him?"* Gammy replied, *"Because he made up rules that not everyone agreed with, and some people were jealous of him.*

Your great grandfather and great grandmother Doyle were good friends with the Kennedys for years. They were good people." Overhearing the conversation from the next room as it unfolded, my father walked into the room, and adding his two cents, saying matter-of-factly, with overt sarcasm, that he, was not a fan of President Kennedy... *"I know lots of people who hate the Kennedys."*

The conversation continued on, but clearly, Dad had a very different, smug and seemingly disdainful opinion of President Kennedy, than Mom and Gammy. At the time, I thought maybe it was because he was not Catholic like Mom and Gammy, but he sounded very sure that he did not agree with them AT ALL. In a chiding sort of way, he talked badly about the whole Kennedy family, saying all sorts of things --so much so, that I wondered if he or his associates knew them personally, somehow.

No, I didn't really understand why Mom thought we needed a

Catholic president or why Dad was so opposed to this particular man being president. All I knew was that they both had very strong views on the topic, and neither would back down. Probably embracing Grammy's views and Mom's sentiments, I left the room feeling a little teary myself, and noticing much tension in the air in our home–and why not? After all, I thought, the president just died! Just several days after President Kennedy was assassinated, I got up in the morning and went downstairs to our playroom to play. It was my parents' anniversary week, so I stopped in at their room to sing, *"Happy Anniversary!"* but no one was there. However, as I passed by the playroom door on the way to the kitchen, I noticed Mom was sitting in the room on a kitchen chair quietly staring at the wall, all by herself. As I peered through the half opened door, I remember seeing Mom sitting motionless, expressionless and staring, mouth open. Her gaze was as if mesmerized by a Turner Classic Movie playing on the big screen. With her short, limp, dark brown hair, frilly top and disheveled, mismatched outfit, she looked to me like some of the homeless people I had seen on the street corners in our small, rural hometown in Upstate New York. Being just 6 years old at the time, I was quite baffled as to what was occurring to my family that day. However, I knew something serious was happening because of the grim expressions on everyone's faces. Howie and Gammy met together in our playroom that day, talking in hushed tones about what to do.

Little did anyone know the long-lasting effects of that fateful day would traumatically impact me for decades to come as Mom did not return from the mental hospital for one and a half years.

That day, I remember standing on a wooden step stool at the front window of our small, rural, three bedroom Cape Cod house with my nose pressed up against the icy glass. I saw the car with her in it roll down our un-shoveled, slippery driveway. The car turned onto the narrow, two lane road in front of our house, and then she vanished into the distance.

By the grace of God, little did I know that she would not return to Upstate New York for a full year and a half! Had I known she would be away so long, I may have lost heart and given up…After Mom left in the car that day, I sat down on the step stool that I had been standing on while watching them place her in the car, crying, wondering to myself about the most basic question many children often ask during vulnerable times: *Who will take care of us kids now that Mom is gone?*

Initially, I was devastated. But, soon, I was consoled by the thought that Dad would be there for my brother and sister and me. Mom had seemed fine to me just days before, then she was catatonic, sitting motionless and dazed in our playroom. It not only felt surreal to see her like that, in my gut I felt for many years that something had gone wrong, very, very wrong.

One of the most curious parts of Mom's becoming catatonic within days of learning about President Kennedy's assassination, was that it was on the week of my parents wedding anniversary. Questions persist, as they swirl around the events surrounding Mom's becoming catatonic. She had been fine just days before. I am certain that the assassination of President Kennedy was not the cause.

Without missing a beat, shortly after Mom was taken away, Howie promptly took us on a two week trip to Arizona, and let us with his sister, Gloria. Before that time, we had never flownany-where that I can recall. When he went to leave us there, I cried and asked him where he was going. He told me he was going to help 'Uncle' Meyer build a big hotel in Las Vegas. Though Aunt Gloria was very good to us kids, I remember sorely missing Dad while he was away on 'business' as he called it. But the timing of the trip always left me with one pressing, unsettling question, even and especially as I grew older and reflected back:

"Why did he have to take the trip so soon after Mom went away to the Seton Institute?"

It all made me wonder if perhaps there was something else that took her down to such a state.

Later, I thought she had looked like she had been drugged. She had been expressionless and almost seemed to be paralyzed sitting in the chair in my playroom for what had seemed like days. The only thing I am sure of is that this condition took her out of commission, and away from us, and I desperately wanted her back.

Silver Lining

So many silver linings in my youth, wherever do I start??? It really is true that everyone has a past, a present, and a future. As you have seen, my childhood was quite traumatic, making it difficult to move on from it at intervals. In fact, I would say that some of the events of my childhood at times have had a haunting effect on my own state of mind and my physical health.

I have consciously chosen to do whatever it takes to live in the present, and have, after five decades, been successful at doing so. As you will see in future chapters, a plethora of unsettling PTSD flashbacks and nightmares have forced me to revisit my childhood trauma through therapy, hence this book. Though I have difficulties with my hands, I am grateful to God for the ability to be able to type on my computer to write and share my story with others.

My silver lining is found in knowing that Jesus is with me, and that many people may be helped by hearing or reading my story. Most of all, I am grateful that Jesus protected me, guided me, and comforted me in my childhood years. Jesus was with me through it all, even when I was in dangerous situations, put in harm's way by my father and his Mob associates. In my adulthood, the Lord provided me with the ability or gift to forgive my parents for their shortcomings and vulnerabilities. Truly, forgiveness is not something I could accomplish on my own. I tried to heal on my own. Due to the intense experiences I had with each of my parents, it has taken many years of prayer, meetings with my priest, and psychotherapy to be able to extend the proverbial olive branch to my mother and father for all that happened in my youth. And in my humanness, though it is imperative for my health and well-being, I sometimes still fall short in being able to forgive them, but I continue to try. For me, it is only possible with Godly intervention. On my own, all bets are off.

But there is a lighter side to my early life. Through the process of therapeutic writing, and many 'ah-hah' and 'déjà vu' moments over the past years from awakenings, corroborative nightmares and flashbacks, I have discovered something I never had for my parents before: compassion and empathy. I feel blest to have come to realize just how much my mother suffered with mental illness, and how it colored her life, relationships, and perspective in every way. She certainly did not have an easy life. In fact, it must have been incredibly hard for Mom living with my father in their early married years, as they lived in, such different worlds. Being a devout old school Catholic, it was terribly hard for Mom being a divorced woman against her will, and a single mother with three children. Living in poverty, she struggled to keep us fed and with a roof over our head, all the while trying not to say anything derogatory about my father. For Mom, living with mental illness eventually cost her marriage, stirred much turmoil and angst with her children, and kept her isolated from enjoying life. I feel so blest to have gained this relatively new understanding of my mom. I am able to remember her in a much kinder way now than ever before.

This compassionate reframing of memories relating to my mother has also been very helpful when looking at my father and his associates. I have had sheer disgust in my heart for his world.

Yet, when I think about him growing up in the Bronx, I take pause now. Once I realized that his Mob associations started when he was very young and he and his family lived in a central Mafia hub in the Bronx, at a time when the Mob was in full sight, it is no wonder that his close associates were who and what they were. He was, in a way, born into the 'Good fella' lifestyle by the location of his birth.

Sure, Howie had a choice as we all do as to what path he would choose. But perhaps he was compelled in some way to walk away from what was good and right and true and embrace the dark side, the seedier way of life. When Howie was just 17 years old, his father left home abruptly and never returned, leaving Howie to support his mother, twin sister and older sister during The Great Depression. Though he had this large responsibility of taking care of his sisters and mother, my Mom often told me Howie was not good to his mother. Many years later, Howie and his two sisters were finally reunited with my grandfather after he resurfaced in his 80's when he went to live in a Masonic Home in Upstate New

York. He had been reportedly living in Hawaii and then Arizona and located by Howie's sisters.

Sometimes a new perspective is what is necessary to forgive someone who has hurt you, and prayer is never wasted and always helpful. I hope praying for my parents has been helpful to them, but I know it has been extremely helpful to me. I have discovered that forgiveness is necessary for good mental and physical health. For me, I realize now that I am on the road to forgiveness whenever I can pray for one who has hurt me. I also *pray fervently and often for my dad's associates by name*, in particular, "Uncle Meyer" Lansky from Saratoga Springs, New York, the "5 families of New York," and their extended families.

CHAPTER 3:
The 'At-Risk' Child

*"God, grant me the serenity to accept the things I cannot change;
The courage to change the things I can,
and the wisdom to know the difference..."*

*"Living one day at a time; enjoying one moment at a time,
Accepting hardships as the pathway to peace,
taking, as He did, this sinful world as it is.
"Not as I would have it;
trusting that He will make all things right*

*If I surrender to His Will;
that I may be reasonably happy in this life,
supremely happy with Him forever in the next. Amen"*

The Serenity Prayer / Reinhold Niebuhr

O riginally, I made three attempts in a year and a half to write down about the childhood trauma that transpired in my youth, and resurfaced in PTSD flashbacks and nightmares, all to no avail.

Each time I fell into clinical depression for a matter of weeks, and was unable to continue.

Perhaps I was just not ready, I thought. However, God's timing is always perfect. Finally, on the fourth try, many traumatic childhood memories came flooding back to my attention, and rather than falling into clinical depression, I was able to prayerfully record them. It has been said that fear and faith cannot coexist. I believe I failed the first three times due to fear. Perhaps I did not feel ready; maybe I was so bogged down with medical issues and overwhelmed at the time.

However, once I realized that God was with me and allowed me to go back so he could heal my childhood memories, I had the strength and confidence to press on.

Particularly in dysfunctional families or families in crisis, it is not uncommon to have a code of silence, as well as, one child who stands out as an 'at-risk child.' In my family, that child was me. The dysfunction may be subtle, primarily only known to close family members, or the dysfunction may be overt, known to many people surrounding the family. It is easy to tell which child it is, by the way that the other family members describe him (or her). No, no one in my family would ever say, *'Adele was the at-risk child in our family.'* Yet the message came through loud and clear.

The child who is described as 'not like the rest of us,' 'the black sheep,' 'a white sheep,'

'precocious,' 'an odd duck,' 'at risk' or 'dancing to her/his own drumbeat' by siblings, parents, neighbors, teachers and/or other family members is often, though not always, what I call the 'lightening-rod child' in a dysfunctional family. This child may also refuse to keep silent about any abuse or wrongful activities within the family either while these activities are happening, or at a later time, despite best efforts by family members to silence them even into in adulthood.

Other common references to the 'lightening-rod child' may include descriptions such as 'the class clown,' 'under-achiever,' 'not working up to her/his potential' or 'my ADHD kid' when the diagnosis has not yet been officially pursued, or professionally made. I have also heard seasoned, loving, weary mothers simply describe at-risk children as 'my one.' Sometimes at-risk children may have ADHD and/or behavior problems and are described in a way that clearly sets them apart from the rest of the family, from their school mates, or other neighborhood children. Sadly, those were the targets of Howie's recruitment efforts, something I discovered many, many years after the fact.

For whatever reason, possibly because of the chaos and mayhem at home, or high-risk children, often go through childhood experiencing significant medical challenges, mental health issues and learning difficulties that go unattended. They may be appropriately or inappropriately labeled as having 'behavior problems.' This, in turn, can initiate or perpetuate the self-fulfilling behavior, social isolation, learning challenges, and the negative connotations ascribed to these children that they may well carry with them throughout life and into adulthood. As these at risk children get older, it is not uncommon for them to turn to drugs or alcohol at a very early age in an effort to self-medicate to try to numb the pain of not being loved or well-connected to their other family members. These young people easily fall through the cracks, sometimes they become truant and develop addictions, and often are unable for various reasons to finish high school. They may become further marginalized as their dysfunctional family issues fade into the background, and they may become known to local law enforcement, as well. Elementary and middle school teachers, social workers, school nurses and pediatricians are in a prime position to be a valuable resource in identifying at-risk children at an early age before this scenario plays out and sidelines their educational process. For the astute observer, the signs are usually there to flag an 'at-risk' child so that they may be helped. The unkempt child, the class clown, the class bully, the class victim, the frequent flyer in the nurse's office, the truant that skips school often, the student that sleeps through class, those who defy authority, even at an early age; children who engage in self-medicating, cutting themselves, or experimenting with street drugs at a very young age long before their peer group and class mates have engaged in these activities. These are just some of the various behaviors that teachers and school nurses might observe in children who are hurting from some sort of untreated childhood trauma at home

These children may have trouble with focusing, learning, sitting in a classroom chair at a desk, getting along with other children, or following rules. They may attach themselves to the adults in their lives that validate their very existence such as teachers, school nurses, a neighbor, or an adult friend of the family. In fact, they may be more comfortable with adults as they seek to replace the attention they do not or cannot receive at home. Many times these children are at increased risk for becoming victims of sexual predators who frequently prey on marginalized children. due to their impulsivity, vulnerable nature and lack of connectedness to their families.

In my own dysfunctional family, I was the at-risk child. I was the focus of my mother's angst, mental illness and wrath, and later realized that my father used me mercilessly, without my knowledge, to help him with his underworld recruitment to build his organization with his 'associates.'

Not until I began having ongoing, repeat PTSD flashbacks and nightmares, and the subsequent writing of this book, did all the pieces of my childhood puzzle begin to come together, and I began to understand the ramifications of Howie's world. I had no idea what he was doing at the time, as I was very young when it started. Each place we went with him, each associate and family we met, was experienced as an adventure unto itself. Because of my youth, I lacked the ability to connect the dots to see the big picture. The pattern spanned over a thirteen year time frame, from when I was about five years old, forward to age eighteen.

Hands down, the best part of remembering my childhood, for me, is that I am now able to pray very specifically for both of my parents, Gina and Howie. I am also able to pray for Howie's 'associates' - those who willingly, or unwittingly, followed him, and all the families that suffered because of their close association with him and his other underworld activities . I believe that my ability to pray for both of my parents is evidence that I have forgiven them. I have also learned that forgiveness does not demand that I also need to forget but rather to find a way to embrace what happened in the past, acknowledge it, to move on with life.

The Unwelcome Visitor

One day, when I was about six years old, my housekeeper, Kay, was sitting in our kitchen listening to her taxi dispatcher radio, smoking cigarettes and drinking coffee while I was playing alone in our playroom. My brother and sister were living with Aunt Eva as Mom was still inpatientat the Elizabeth Seton Institute where she stayed for a year and a half. I heard a man, one of Kay's taxi drivers, come into the house asking for me. He talked briefly with Kay, then came in the playroom, grabbed me and took me upstairs to my bedroom.

I do not know for sure how he got past Kay, but he did. He had graying hair and smelled bad, like he smoked too many cigarettes and he drank alcohol for breakfast. Kay had to hear my blood curdling screams for help, as it was a very small house and I was not one to be quiet in the face of danger. When we got upstairs to my room, he threw me on my bed and sexually assaulted me as I screamed for help to no avail.

I do not remember exactly what happened after that, except there was a significant struggle. I must have put up a good fight, as his fist went through the wall above my bed, leaving a fist-size hole in the wall. The next thing I remember is that he got up, pulled his pants up, and ran down stairs.

I ran after him yelling "Help! Help!" Kay never acknowledged my screams or came to my rescue, despite my unceasing calls for help, but as he left the house, the unwelcome visitor threw money at the housekeeper, Kay, got into his taxi and drove away down the driveway. I was absolutely devastated with nowhere to turn for consolation, but to Jesus, the one I always turned to in times of need.

Shaking, and crying hard by myself, I prayed unceasingly that it would never happen to me again.

But I was very afraid he would return. It is highly likely that Kay did not defend me for a reason.

I watched her accept his money that day after the sexual assault, and I went back up to my room and continued to cry a bucket of tears into my pillow.

Who was that man, and why was he here in our house and in my bedroom? Kay definitely knew him as she had let him in. Did Dad know about him coming in our house and trying to hurt me? My young mind was racing, and after I stopped crying, I was incensed. Every emotion seemed to sweep over me in the aftermath, but I was frozen and did not tell anybody about it right away.

After all, who did I have to tell???

When Dad finally came home, I tried to tell him, but felt he did not hear me and it all seemed to fall on deaf ears. At the time, I felt so violated, so humiliated, so ashamed, that I just wanted to forget the whole thing forever. I buried the memory as deeply as possible. To this day, I will never know if Dad knew about the man in my bedroom who sexually assaulted me. It was never clear what he was supposed to be doing there that day. I tried desperately to tell my father what had happened to me, but it was as if he could not hear me. As I look back over what happened, I feel better knowing that I fought hard to protect what belonged to me and me alone.

Finally, about 50 years later I was in therapy with a very caring and kind therapist who was so helpful when I told her the sexual assault that had happened some five decades before, and I was able to work through it at last! As for the large hole in the wall above my bed, no one seemed to notice for many months, despite my pleas for my dad to fix it. Much later, after my mother's return home, my parents asked me why I had damaged the wall and I was admonished for causing it. The hole in the wall occurred when the man's fist went through the dry wall during the sexual assault. Again, to no avail I tried to tell both of them what happened, and I was accused of having a big imagination. No one ever did fix the hole in my wall above my bed. I guess with all that was going on at home at the time, it was a small, insignificant thing to them, but it was a constant reminder to me. After that fateful day, I experienced night terrors and sleep walking for years, but never received therapy in my childhood to help me deal with what had happened.

Yes, there were definitely deep and lasting wounds from what happened. It certainly seemed that Kay assisted the man by ignoring me pleas and not responding to my calls for help, and she did, after all, accept his money. Did Howie set me up? I will never know. All I know for sure is that though I had no real words, no language to describe what happened to me that day in my own bed with absolutely no one to tell, I buried the memory deep inside, in hopes it wouldn't bother me ever again. I just tried to get on with living and to forget the whole thing. I had no idea, as years passed by, how that experience would fester like a gaping wound, and affect me emotionally, mentally, physically, and spiritually, and in that way, be an ongoing source of torment, and angst in my mind, body, and soul.

From that day forward, for years, even as my parents called me Bright Eyes, I felt so humiliated, violated, ashamed and truly broken, but I also felt it was my job to try to keep the peace at home and not muddy the waters. From that day forward I had such conflicting feelings about what happened and what should have been done about it. I lived with a shrapnel wound in my soul that would not heal.

Today, however, I believe what happened is called child sex trafficking, and it is a serious felony with years of jail time. Whether it was Kay's own doing, or Howie's licentiousness, I will never know. I have, however, written it all down and escorted it, and evicted it, out of my conscious being. With confidence I can say, I no longer hold this soul-shattering event in my heart, for it is now secret no more! And I am victim no more. I have long ago forgiven Kay, the unwelcome stranger, and my parents, as well, as I am able to pray for them all! It is only with God's help I have been able to forgive.

Mom's Homecoming

A year and a half later, in the spring of 1964 when I was seven years old, Mom was discharged from the St. Elizabeth Seton Institute. Her discharge dovetailed with the time when the trend was to 'de-institutionalize' the mentally ill and discharge them home or to the streets. The day of her discharge from the mental institution,

Howie had someone meet her upon her arrival at the airport and serve her with separation papers.

Though he must have conferred with her doctors before discharge, Howie did not allow Mom to come home. In her fragile mental state, fresh out of the mental institution, she was instantly homeless from the time the plane landed and she was served papers. There was nothing she could do at the time to fight back.

Thank God my grandmother, Gammy, was with her that day as she was still quite fragile from her long hospitalization. Dad had custody of us kids for a while, then that arrangement was reversed, and, despite the fact that Mom chose to be un-medicated for her mental illness, she was given custody of us three kids for the duration of our childhoods. After her return from Seton, Mom was extremely difficult to live with as she was emotionally distraught, chronically agitated, and displayed raging anger most of the time. From what Mom later told me when I was old enough to understand, she suffered with and was hospitalized in the 60's at Seton with severe major depression and Obsessive Compulsive Disorder, or OCD. Years later, after describing her behavior to my therapist, I was told that due to her earlier catatonic state, agitation and paranoia were most likely due to schizophrenia.

As the years marched on, Mom refused all psychiatric help and medication. It was all just part of her mental illness, but her choices made it really hard to live together as a family. Living with her was difficult beyond measure. I believe Mom was a tormented woman unable to control her cruelty, her irritability, her agitation, her 'I love you/I hate you' cycling, and uncontrolled rages, and her most unusual repetitive activities from her obsessive compulsive disorder (OCD) made it difficult to be a family. But we kids loved her dearly, all the same. Clearly, I hated her cruelty, and the embarrassment of living with a Mother who was acutely mentally ill.

However, I tried to love her to the best of my ability and help her wherever I could, though it felt like a futile effort. The hard truth is, it's almost impossible to help someone who is cruel, psychotic, and irrational most of the time who rejects all help.

The Butterfly

When I was about 9 years old, I happened upon a beautiful butterfly with a broken wing in our front yard in Upstate New York. With all the desire of a nurse in training, I picked up the butterfly and placed it in an old shoebox, and added twigs, grass, and an old bottle cap filled with water for extra measure. I checked on my little butterfly friend about 3 times a day, hoping that it's colorful wing would heal enough for it to fly again one day soon.

Day after day, I nurtured it along, until one day, I heard it flapping its wings in the home made little habitat I had prepared, and it was clearly time to see if it could fly again. Opening the lid to peek in, I could see both wings fluttering and trusted the time had come to let it go. Filled with both excitement and ambivalence, I took the small shoebox over to the little hill between our house and our neighbor's house. Carefully, I placed my hand inside the box until the butterfly was squarely on my outstretched forefinger. Then I lifted the top of the box and stood up, as the butterfly stayed on my finger!

With a few tears, a little nudge and some encouraging words, my butterfly friend went flying off across between yards. Then something unexpected happened. The butterfly circled a tree and started to come back towards me!

Surely it would turn and fly away, I thought, but it did not. My beautiful, healed butterfly continued to come towards me. Full of surprise, anticipation, and wondering what would happen next, I lifted my forefinger up for it to land on just in case…and it did!

I will never really know how it happened that day that my little butterfly friend returned to me and landed right on my forefinger, but I can tell you I considered it, and still do, nothing short of serendipity—A God wink. In my young mind, it was probably the first time I was aware of a God-happening, a sort of albeit small, miracle in my life. I wondered if that was how the 'Holy Spirit' my mother had told me about worked. Thinking about the way I found it, and the wing healing with a little help, I somehow found myself thinking that that must be how God worked in our lives, that He takes our brokenness and transforms it into blessings. This much I do know.

That little butterfly gave me hope, and for that I was eternally grateful! Hope for my difficult life, hope that I was no longer alone in my struggles, and hope in my ability to fulfill my dream to become a registered nurse one day. Who could think that God could profoundly, spiritually touch and change a young life for the better through a wounded butterfly!

Shasta & the 'Family Reunion'

One day, when I was about 11 years old, while my siblings and I were visiting Dad's older cousin, Uncle John in New Jersey, I overheard him say emphatically to my Dad: "Howie!

I want you to get the whole family together! Everybody! We are getting a place near Atlantic City, and I want everyone there!" Naively thinking we were having a family reunion, I could hardly wait to tell my brother and sister about our upcoming family reunion and the opportunity to meet more of our cousins and extended family. Much later, I learned that the meeting was called because the boss of the Bonanno Family, 'Joe Bananas,' was missing, and no one knew where he was. It seemed from what Dad said that they needed to find him and/or replace him quickly.

The day finally arrived, and we traveled to the beach house just outside of Atlantic City. Shortly upon arrival, my sister and brother quickly got in their swim suits and headed for the beach before I was ready, so I stayed behind trusting that my dad would take me to the beach soon afterwards. As a precocious young child, I was persistently by Dad's side whenever possible.

With elbows propped up on the table, hands under my chin during meetings with his 'associates,' and even while he was gambling and drinking, I presented Dad with quite a challenge, especially when he was 'doing business,' as his mantra was 'Children should be seen and not heard.' I suppose I didn't get that particular memo in my youth, but my sister told me many years later about it. To my great surprise, shortly after my siblings left to walk to the beach, about a dozen rough looking strangers, men of all ages, showed up and stood in formation, hands at their sides, before my Dad and Uncle John for roll call, followed by a meeting. I remember they were all ages and sizes, and I recognized two of them as people Dad had met with while I was with him. I remember thinking, as my Dad took roll-call, my Dad must be the leader and, *"Who are these men, and what are they doing at our family reunion?"*

In reality, they were the reason we were there at the beach house in the first place. They needed to get a plan and find a replacement for family boss, Joe Bonanno, who they called "Joe Bananas," who had gone missing. As they began roll-call, and then to talk 'business,' one of the men at the small table bobbed his head in my direction saying in a gravelly, loud voice, *"Hey Howie! What about Ears?"*

Without missing a beat, Dad said, *"I'll take care of it!"*

Then, Dad shouted emphatically, *"Somebody get Adele a Shasta!"*

One of the men brought me a Shasta soda right away. Being the only child there, and feeling quite special, I drank the Shasta soda straight away, and had no memory for what happened after that, except to say we were there for a about a week, and I never did get to the beach or get to hang out with my siblings and cousins. At the end of the week, my siblings talked about all the fun they had, and I had no memory whatsoever of ever having gone to the beach with them.

Not sure what kind of person would do such a thing to a child, but as a nurse, my best guess is that someone apparently slipped rufinol or something like it into the Shasta soda. rufinol, also known as the date rape drug that allows a person to function, but erases all memory for what occurs while under the influence. Needless to say, that may be the reason for my earlier long term memory loss for many of the meetings I attended with Howie, and for memories of my youth at-large, from about age 5 to 18.

Days later, when Howie came to tell me it was time to go home, I remember still feelinggroggy and nauseas, but had no memory for the week long 'vacation.' It is noteworthy that after that week, wherever and whenever I went with Howie by myself to New Jersey or New York City, I was usually offered a Shasta soda, which became my nickname with his 'business associates' whenever we visited them.

No, I will probably never know why Dad always seemed to enter establishments via the back or side door, or why he had so many friends and associates who did the same thing. Even when he reunited with his father whom he hadn't seen since he was 17 when he mysteriously left his family some four decades earlier, he had someone drive grandpa in a golf cart to the back fence of the spacious Masonic Home in Utica, New York to meet us, rather than entering through the front door. I will never understand why he always seemed to be looking over his shoulder, and avoiding the law wherever we went with him, or why he took us to 'The Block,' in Baltimore City, stopping to get a drink at a well-known show bar while we three kids patiently waited outside the establishment on the sidewalk amongst the sordid characters waiting to go in, or why he was fascinated by Baltimore legend Blaze Starr. I will probably never fully know why he was always holding meetings with his 'associates' wherever he went, many he had known since his youth in the Bronx, and the service, and others from Upstate New York, New Jersey, Washington, DC and across Maryland. Many of his closest 'associates' were first and second generation Italian immigrants, usually with Sicilian background, and some others from countries all over the globe, including Italy, the United Kingdom, Poland, Cuba, Iran, Syria, and Saudi Arabia. He seemed to focus his efforts on recruiting people from large families.

Over the years, Howie often held meetings in various locations, including ethnic restaurants like Grimaldi's in Upstate New York, Cagney's, Giovanni's, Little Italy in Baltimore, and even the Greek restaurant, the Acropolis, in Baltimore, talking most about Luigi (Meyer Lansky), 'The Syndicate,' 'The Sicilians,' 'the Cosa Nostra,' 'The Commission,' the governing body of the 5 families of New York, Jimmy Hoffa and the Teamsters Union, all the while playing cards and drinking with his compadres as I/we kids waited outside for him to finish. They also talked about trafficking and imports and exports, bringing people from Cuba into the US, casinos and the 'entertainment business.' These conversations were highly reflective of the diversification of their activities and the close connection between the Cosa Nostra, the Italian Mafia, and the American Mafia, also known as the Meyer Lansky's Syndicate. In essence, Dad and 'Uncle' Meyer worked together with both organizations to accomplish their sordid goals. Even in my teens, while repeatedly witnessing these underworld conversations and meetings, I was unable to 'connect the dots' until much, much later.

What I do know is that later in my life, I realized that Dad's conversations that I witnessed with many of his closest associates in the early to mid-70's, told me all I needed to know about him once I connected the dots in my adult years. Though Mom seemed to know precious little about Dad's 'business activities' she wisely often said: *"Birds of a Feather Really Do Flock Together!"* I never really got the sense that Mom had a firm understanding of dad's double life, his activities, and his actual relationships with his associates. There was certainly no business partnership in their marriage. My mother was a smart and intuitive soul. Surely she must have had some idea as the years pressed on as to some of his activities. The only time I think Mom ever connected the dots was when she came to me one day when my sister was away at college and told me, *"I'm afraid your father is in a little bit of trouble."* I was in high school at the time, and no matter how hard I pressed her for more information, she refused to divulge what it was about.

During the early years of my childhood, Howie was a brilliant, energetic bow-tie wearing mechanical engineer working in Upstate New York. As far as I know, he left his job as a mechanical engineer when I was about 12 years old. This was close to the time my parents divorced in 1969 while we were still in Upstate New York. Later, after we moved with Mom to the DC area, he seemed to have changed his career, to what I do not know.

There is an old saying: Show me your friends and I will tell you who you are. This statement is certainly relevant to my father. Looking back, I suppose the many conversations I overheard while with my Dad and his Mob associates told more of the story than I ever really wanted to know in my youth. However, I was unable to connect the dots for decades, as many seemingly random pieces of the puzzle began to fall into place. I was in my late 40's and early 50's when it all came flooding back to me as I began to heal from PTSD.

In our family, my siblings and I had an unspoken understanding, a silence, about our life together and about our parents, so I was unable to share my quest and thirst for needing to understand Howie's world. My siblings simply seemed to have no interest in answering the questions that I held close. Interestingly, as I became an adult, Howie's world unraveled before me. I discovered the reality of his life one puzzle piece at a time through people who knew him, and a seemingly endless series of repeat PTSD flashbacks, particularly while living in the Baltimore metro area. However, though Howie became far more active in the Mob, and open with me about his 'double life.' Not sure why, but my siblings have yet to connect the dots, and nor do they seem to have the desire to do so.

As a very young girl, and through the end of high school, I remember Dad was often leading meetings with his associates everywhere we went about what I simply called, politics and business. With his rough-cut, hard drinking, cigarette and cigar smoking New York and New Jersey 'associates,' he most often talked in front of me about, 'Luigi [Uncle Meyer]' 'The Italians' 'The Sicilians,' 'Cosa Nostra,' 'The Syndicate,' 'Our Thing,' 'The Rackets,' 'Hoffa and the Teamsters Union,' 'The Chicago Outfit,' and casinos in Las Vegas and Atlantic City.

They talked about 'The Commission,' the governing body of the New York/New Jersey 'Syndicate,' bringing people into the 'entertainment industry,' whatever that meant, 'trafficking'

(of what or whom I do not know), and, of course, Luigi, Meyer Lansky, Dad's mentor. They also talked about his other longtime 'business associates,' Cody, Roy, Vito, Pajamas, union boss Jimmy Hoffa, Giancana, Bonanno, Tony, Adonis, Carlo and Manny Gambino, John G. and Sammy, and Joe Z. the Bookie, many of whom I met in my early childhood in New Jersey and New York, and again, later in my life. To my recollection, Howie's 'business associates' that I met when my siblings were living with my aunt when I was around 6 years old were mostly Sicilian Italians or Sicilian Americans. I met many of those same associates again in the Baltimore metro area while I was in middle school and high school when Howie openly introduced me to his world, and again later in adulthood.

Howie also talked with his associates about finding new and creative ways to bring people into the country across the Canadian and Mexican borders, and especially by boat from Cuba into Florida. He often talked of Ponzi money-making schemes, and ways to collect money from people and businesses, something my father referred to as graft. To my dismay, much later I learned that graft was a form of extortion, accomplished by forcibly taking money from people, a substantial percentage of the money others earned through their hard work. As a young child, I witnessed the banter between my father and his gruff, pinky-ringed associates with much curiosity, as they had developed their own slang language to secretly describe their activities.

This code became more prevalent and discernable for me with each passing year, especially from middle school forward.

I clearly remember some of the places we went, pieces of conversations I overheard, and nicknames of many of the associates Dad encountered who were, at the time, part of his illicit activities. It took me many decades before I could connect the dots, in part, because they were covert about their real names, often using nicknames, and localities. I lacked the understanding to fully embrace the evil in which he was involved. Actually, I did not realize that they often spoke in code until I was in college. At that point, I quickly came to understand that others could not comprehend some of my father's 'common' slang that I had incorporated into my own language. I had learned many terms that I had heard often in my youth, while spending time with Dad and his card-playing, hard drinking 'business associates.'

Fast Forward

It is noteworthy that I had profound learning problems in my youth, and some still exist today.

Even as I was struggling to learn to read and write until the end of the 4th grade, I was also in a 'high risk' group at school for years, but no one seemed to make a connection with my parents, or my home life. In fact, my parents seemed distant and uninformed of my learning problems in school.

This was long before we knew so much about learning disabilities like dyslexia, and the like. The connection between untreated childhood trauma, learning issues, and some auto-immune and neurological infirmities later in life is a curious one; one that begs for more controlled medical research.

Unable to read and write until the end of the fourth grade, I suppose to my detriment, I had endured too much, seen too much, and heard too much, at too young an age, from Gina's and Howie's worlds. One day in the 4th grade, I was removed from my class and placed in a special education program. However, I refused to sit in the seat. At that point, I became a behavior problem for the principal. My parents were never called in as far as I know. I had to meet with my teacher and the principal and it was decided I could return to my regular class room with the room mother, who mentored me in reading. Finally, after 2-3 months of one-on-one instruction, I was finally on my way! Though I never did get held back a grade, my reading comprehension continued to be a significant issue for me all throughout school and into college, but I was always able to get by in school.

HOMELESS IN THE NEW YORK

In 1969, when I was about 11 years old, we became homeless after my parents divorced. In her grief, Mom prematurely sold the house, and we had nowhere to go. We had precious little money, as Howie had not paid taxes on the house in years, so the money from the house paid the taxes.

We were forced to live in a series of one room, low budget motels with Mom, without food or transportation, from January until June for about 5 months until school was out for the summer.

We survived on donuts and water from the local diner. In actuality, we were homeless and migratory, going from one motel to another as we were repeatedly evicted for not being able to pay for the room the 4 of us all shared. Complaining was not allowed, and Mom was really in a fragile paranoid state.

Mom tried to put a happy face on our situation, and I tried my level best to believe her when she called it 'an adventure.' Interestingly, Howie continued to come on weekends to take us places where he met with his compadres. I remember asking him if we could live with him, as he and his girlfriend lived about a mile away. Without any real explanation, he repeatedly told me that it was *just the way it was.* To my knowledge, he did nothing to help our plight. All I wanted to do was find a place to live, have access to real food, and plenty of it, and put the nightmare behind me. I would have been content to have been adopted by another, higher functioning family!

That winter, my brother and I walked two miles together each way, to and from school, in the blustery Upstate New York cold weather and snow without boots, gloves, and with only light jackets and layered clothes. By the time we got to school each day, we were hungry, wet and frozen to the core from the bitter cold weather and waist high Upstate New York snow. Without snow boots, we became adept at covering our shoes with plastic bread bags attached with rubber bands to keep them in place. Hunger and being cold became commonplace that winter, as meals were not a part of our daily routine at the motel due to lack of funds.

That year, when summer came, and with great relief school ended, we moved from Upstate New York to Takoma Park, Maryland to be near my mother's sister, Aunt Eva in Bethesda, Maryland.

Howie reportedly stayed behind in Upstate New York with his other family, that is, his girlfriend and her daughter. We pressed on to build a new life with my mother, near Aunt Eva, and Gammy continued to come and try to help when Mom was deeply psychotic, but it certainly wasn't easy for them either.

I remember well crying, and praying, and asking God how he could possibly allow us to be homeless, and live with Mom, as she was cruel and frail. Depending on her was difficult and scary as her behavior was so erratic. I never really knew if my mother loved or hated me. Hoping against hope, I prayed that someone would find our little family and save us kids from the poverty, turmoil and torment which was our daily life. Though I begged God for a new family and a warm home, that prayer seemed to go unanswered.

In my optimistic 12 year old mind, I hoped that perhaps my Dad would be able and willing to save us from Mom's reach. Yet he hardly seemed to notice our plight despite my repeated heartfelt pleas. Howie had another family as he lived with his longtime girlfriend whom he had moved into town with, and her daughter. Yes, he came and took us three kids to fun places on the weekends, and I enjoyed the respite from being homeless with Mom, but the reality was we were very hungry and homeless, and he had left for good and had a new life. It was time to face it: he was never going to be someone I could depend on. He was never coming back. I was angry with him, and loathed his aloofness and coldness, but I just had to accept the fact he was a dead beat dad, which is why I started referring to him, of course not to his face, as 'Good Time Charlie.'

For me, it was a lot to digest, but something told me I just needed to get over my angst and move on as best I could. After tossing the situation around in my mind over and over, I realized that our circumstances were awful, but temporary, and that Jesus alone would give us whatever we needed to sustain us. This was probably the first time I began to pray to God fervently and recognized that Father God had so much more to offer me in my life than my dad ever could. After that realization, I asked Jesus for whatever we needed with renewed confidence and trust. After all, for years I had tried in so many ways to get my father to help us to no avail. In my young mind I reasoned, what did I have to lose?

I guess in a way I was at a point of testing God's metal. So I would pray and ask for the basic things we needed, food, shelter, clothing, then wait and see what happened. A lot of the time nothing happened, but I just kept asking him to help us. I felt abandoned, rejected, and neglected by his seeming indifference to our plight. Historically, my family often talked about the 'squeaky wheel getting the grease.' That was the paradigm for my prayer 'test.' No, there were usually no instant results; but I felt better just knowing that I had given it to God, asking for what I needed to the One whom I had heard could do anything. Somehow, asking Father God for what we needed made me feel better.

Silver Lining

*"Consider it pure joy, my brothers and sisters,
whenever you face trials of many kinds,
because you know that the testing of your faith produces perseverance."*

James 1:2-3

Perseverance...I've got that! I truly believe that Jesus himself shielded me from succumbing to my mother's wrath and from the dangers of Howie's world until the time was just right. This occurred in my fifties. How did I know when the time was right? Well, for the first time, I became able to process truths from my past without lapsing into depression, crying, ruminating, becoming fearful, or condemnation of myself or my parents, as I struggled to reach for forgiveness. For me, I knew my time had come to forgive when I began to pity their plights, Mom with her mental illness, and Howie with his activities and his despotic Mob associates, and pray for them both.

My mother likely knew about some of Howie's earlier 'Mob activities,' as she sometimes talked about Howie and his associates to me as I grew older. However, it seemed she could not face it all and she succumbed to mental illness, catatonia in fact, at about the age of 41 when she was admitted into the mental institution. I have often wondered if what happened to Mom was organic or something else. Perhaps, like Shakespeare's Lady Macbeth, she saw something that made her develop OCD. I know that early in my life, she liked to believe the best in people.

Howie's Mob activities would have been really tough for her to digest—If not impossible.

One thing I do know. Many in the Mob had wives that were "partners," yet some were willing to ignore their husband's Mob activities. I believe that my mother was the latter.

Today I am past the point of anger, judgment, condemnation, and despair. Rather, I have chosen to put each aside to spend my time and energy more positively, praying for those in most need of God's mercy; those souls who have no one to pray for them. In this way, I am free and unencumbered to pray fervently and by name for those I met so long ago in Howie's world.

I have learned a lot about compassion along the way. There are no perfect people, myself included. I am free to pray for the Mom and Howie, the 'Five families of New York' and all their many compadres, sympathizers, and extended family members. I am free to look on Gina's life and Howie's World, through the eyes of compassion… There but for the grace of God, go I…

Though I have endured much, I truly believe that Jesus is, and has been, with me throughout my life. Long gone is the shame and indignation I experienced for decades regarding my sense that I was born into the wrong family; that God had made a mistake when He placed me in my family of origin. Long gone are the days when I used to pray that someone would learn of our plight and adopt me and my siblings out of my mother's care. Gone are the days when I felt I would crumble if I really understood who my father was and what he really did. Yes, all those feelings have faded away into the past.

Today, I find it is a divine privilege to pray for those in my life who are in most need of God's mercy, compassion and love, and to recognize that the human condition is one riddled with faults and mistakes. The hard truth is that neither of my parents were capable of love. Yet who really has the capacity to truly love others unconditionally as God loves us? Holding another in contempt is always a bad idea, as it has been said that *"when you point a finger at someone, there are four pointing back at you."* Best of all, I have been able to pray for both of them; which for me, is a solid act of forgiveness.

By the grace of God, for the glory of God, I have finally been able to embrace healing in the face of adversity. Now I clearly recognize that fear and faith cannot coexist; neither can we move along in our own lives if we refuse to forgive others their trespasses. I have chosen to live a hope-filled and joy-filled life. In truth, the Bible says that God forgives us as we forgive others.

At last, the trials I have endured as an 'At-Risk Child' can bear good fruit, the fruit of compassion, as I have grown exponentially in my ability to forgive and grown in patience and persistence. In as much as it has been said that *underneath every pile of anger is a mound of sadness,* I am ever so grateful to God that He is, through Jesus Christ the Great Healer and Comforter, healing me from the inside out! He has effectively healed my fears, my sadness; and my deep feelings of shame, rejection, and abandonment.

CHAPTER 4:
Naming and Claiming Childhood Trauma

*"There is a time for everything
and a season for every activity under the heavens..."*

*a time to be born and a time to die,
a time to plant and a time to uproot,
a time to kill and a time to heal,
a time to tear down and a time to build,
a time to weep and a time to laugh,
a time to mourn and a time to dance,
a time to scatter stones and a time to gather them,
a time to embrace and
a time to refrain from embracing,
a time to search and a time to give up,
a time to keep and a time to throw away,
a time to tear and a time to mend,
a time to be silent and a time to speak,
a time to love and a time to hate,
a time for war and a time for peace."*

Ecclesiastes 3:1-8

The Captive Teen Years

Circa 1971, when I was in middle school, Howie moved to the Baltimore metro area to Middle River, Maryland from Utica, New York leaving his other family behind saying he wanted to be closer to us kids. He would drive down to our apartment, and pick us up for weekend visits from Takoma Park, Maryland where we lived on his assigned weekends. He would take us to places where he consistently held informal 'meetings' at people's homes in the Baltimore Metro area in fields, at spelunking caves in Harper's Ferry, West Virginia, cliff climbing, wherever. His M.O. was to send us off to do something fun as a sort of diversion, so he could privately 'talk business' with his associates who seemed to repeatedly just show up wherever we went. Not being athletic or an adventurous hiker, I often stayed behind with him and his 'associates' during his 'meetings.'

After my parents divorced, through middle and high school, while living with Mom in Takoma Park, Maryland near Aunt Eva, money for clothing, blankets and food in our home were rare commodities. In fact, hunger was a constant companion. With ice on the inside of our windows in the winter, we used our winter coats as extra blankets at night, and had few clothes and little food was available. Yes, poverty was in full bloom in our home while living with Mom. Her idea of cooking a meal was making peanut butter and jelly sandwiches, cereal, or heating an open can of Spaghettio's directly on the open gas flame of our stove!

Dealing daily with poverty, cold and hunger were always in the forefront of my mind, and just became a part of life. Mom was sick physically and psychotic most of the time, and trying her level best just to survive living with untreated mental illness, let alone struggling to raise 3 children as a single mother. Yet, no matter how tough it was at home with Mom and her agitation and cruelty, I always knew instinctively in my heart, that I could step away from her when I needed to for survival, but I could never walk away from her for good…and I never did. I believed that one day I would be free of my mother's constant berating and blaming me for the break-up of her marriage to my father, something I never really understood. I was grounded in my room for months at a time in both middle and high school for getting caught smoking cigarettes or being sassy. Rarely, if ever, was I allowed to attend social events such as high school football games or other school sports or school dances other than homecoming and the prom. Only Catholic Church Catholic Youth Organization (CYO) events were allowed. There were whole summers at a time —from June to September-- when I was 'incarcerated' by Mom this way through middle school and high school, unable to use the phone to connect with friends, or leave my room except for meals. The isolation was beyond difficult. Yet my brother and sister were allowed to do a lot more, go places with friends, and were rarely, if ever, grounded like I was. They had a lot more freedom to go out with friends, etc. It is ironic that during many summers of my 'captivity,' I was only allowed to go with Howie on his visitation weekends and to church. Not surprisingly, these periods of 'incarceration' were the result of talking back to my mother, or smoking cigarettes, which seemed to fuel my mother's mental illness and her unfairly, overtly holding me responsible for her marital break-up.

One of the ways I dealt with these long periods of 'incarceration' was by reading the Holy Bible.

The problem was that my mother believed that only a Catholic priest could read the Bible and interpret Scripture, and I was not allowed to have one or read it. So I obtained a Good News Bible, and hid it under my bed! Whenever I got sad or anxious, I would pull it out from under my bed and read the Psalms, Philippians, or Ephesians or the book of Matthew for solace. Without the Bible, my life would have been much more difficult. With the Bible, I received the life-giving encouragement I needed to press on. However, the abuse at home with Mom, for me, was ongoing, intense, unrelenting, and escalating. Throughout high school and middle school, my mother would often come and wake me up on school nights between 10:00pm and 11:00pm, ranting abusively sometimes until 2:00A.M. telling me how she was sorry I was ever born. The experience was so intense and detrimental to me, causing sleep deprivation and sleeping during classes, that the school nurse helped me get one period a day in school where they reserved a cot for me to sleep during school. Ultimately, the school did nothing else as they waited for me to get the nerve to submit paperwork they gave me to go into foster care, something I simply could not bring myself to do.

My mother's seemingly non-stop cruelty towards me evolved exponentially after my sister went away to college in 1971. Before that time, I had not realized all my sister did to help my mother emotionally stay on keel. She was, in essence, Mom's handler. After she was gone, my mother lost her direction and no longer had a sounding board to help her stay on track. It seemed that once my sister left for college, Mom rapidly became psychotic most of the time. At the same time my Dad also accelerated his Mob 'activities,' 'diversified' his 'business,' expanded his recruitment efforts, and multiplied his associates while overtly introducing me to his world. It was at this point that he reintroduced me to his Sicilian connections and the inner workings of his double life with Meyer Lansky and the Mob.

According to my research, this same time period coincided with the Gambino family's recruitment period in the 70's, which may explain a lot. He introduced me to boss Carlo Gambino.

Some families, like my own, are so chaotic that they don't notice overt changes in behavior or turn away from and avoid dealing with feelings of one who is hurting from abuse or neglect, abandonment or rejection. In my family, both with my parents and siblings, we had three unspoken codes of silence, and in essence, to express emotion was unacceptable and scorned.

Our family codes of silence included:

1. Don't tell Mom anything about where we went and what we did with Dad.
2. Don't tell anyone outside of our family about our family dysfunction, our poverty, or Mom's mental illness, or we would be separated and never see each other again.
3. Don't talk among ourselves about our home life; just deal with

it as best you can the un-spoken rule was every child for him/herself.

Actually, while I was growing up in my mother's apartment in Takoma Park, Maryland, I was very private with my peers; careful not to bring middle school or high school friends over lest they see the poverty and dysfunctional family dynamics that I endured living with Mom. For many years throughout my youth, I tried desperately to hide and 'normalize' my early childhood life, but was eventually unable to do so. Though I did not have many friends outside of school, I tried to present my life to others as ordinary, when it was anything but. I think that is partly why I resisted getting help for my depression. I didn't want anyone to know the depth of the pain I harbored inside, even and especially in my middle school and high school years.

As the "At-Risk Child" in our dysfunctional family, my experience and memories were anything but carefree as I was targeted by both of my parents for different reasons. In the recesses of my room, I cried long, hard and often about innocence lost, and being unloved and unlovable. I used to dream of what a happy family experience might look like. And, I prayed that Jesus would heal my family and my inner wounds. When I reached adulthood I still needed professional help from a psychotherapist along with medication from a psychiatrist. These resources eventually allowed me to get on with living to begin to heal my own mind-body-connection. Perhaps finding help WAS the answer to my fervent prayers.

For decades, whenever the topic would come up about my parents or my childhood, I would freeze like a deer in the head lights, as overwhelming, negative feelings would sweep over me.

Often, I changed the subject to avoid having to deal with questions as I lacked the strength to share my family experiences. Questions about my family elicited powerful and uncomfortable emotional and physiological changes. Discussing them produced visceral, gut-wrenching feelings of anger, anguish, fear, guilt, and shame. As I reflect back I realize that these feelings were important clues to understanding my own mind-body-spirit connection.

It is also noteworthy that I was the only one of the three of us privy to the content of Howie's meetings with his closest associates. Precocious from an early age, I was fascinated by my father's life and his often brash but kind associates, and he did not usher me away when they met and I was with him at his side. In fact, he often chose me out of the three of us to accompany him to drive to meetings in New York and New Jersey from the age of four or five when we lived in Utica, New York. Later, I accompanied him to frequent Mob meetings in the Baltimore areas for 5 years, from age 13 to 18 when my sister stopped coming on Dad's visits.

In my middle school and high school years, Howie, went through many times where he spent our weekend visits with just me in tow. During that time, he took me on 'business' meetings with his associates and also engaged in debates at the local Unitarian Universalist Society in Towson, Maryland, trying to *disprove the existence of God*—something he and I debated often and fervently. Much to Howie's chagrin. it became commonplace for me to publicly counter his rhetoric there, as I would stand up, when he was finished with his oration, and refute the negative things he had to say about God.

Needless to say, weekends with Howie were an interesting time once my sister left for college.

My sister was the stabilizing factor in our family, and once she left for college, she was sorely missed by all, as she had acted like a buffer for me, often protecting me from the blunt force of Mom's cruelty. In essence, both of my parents depended on her to be the source of reason; a logical sounding board, of sorts. Without her, our family was careening out of control as my sister had become the mother in our family. With a growing interest in building his Syndicate/American Mafia/Mob organization' with an eclectic, tough guy cast of international characters from Sicily, Italy, Cuba, Puerto Rico, Iran, Syria, Russia, Saudi Arabia, the UK, etc..., Howie was like a man on a mission—what mission I do not know--as he drove his brown Nova to random places both in and out of state on our weekend visits, driving at a manic pace across Maryland, Washington, D.C., Virginia, Delaware, West Virginia, Pennsylvania, sometimes all in one day. We usually ended up in a certain locality in Maryland an hour and a half from where we lived with my mother. Because of this, I was never really sure where we were as there were few signs at that time and he was secretive about where we went. For some reason his favorite place seemed to be in the Baltimore metro area about 30 minutes from where he lived in Middle River, Maryland. The Baltimore metro area is where he took me most often on our weekends, and where I later re-met some of his New York and New Jersey associates and their families again as an adult in the early to mid-80's when my husband and I unknowingly, and unwittingly, moved into the area near where he had held many of his meetings in the 70's.

David and The 'Age of Freedom'

Three years older than me, I missed my sister dearly when she went away to college, as she had held the mother role in our extremely, dysfunctional family. However, in my way of thinking, I thought that if I could just hold on until I was 18 years old to leave home, I would be free. In essence, I could see a light at the end of the darkness I had lived in for so long. In my mind, I believed that after I became an adult at 18, Howie's associates would never have the opportunity again to violate me, and I could walk away from my mother's torment.

At the age of 14, I met a man named David, and [thought I] had fallen in love. Though my mother was justly against the relationship because as he was 7 years older than me [21 years old], the relationship spanned 5 years, having met him at the nursing home where I was a candy striper, and he was a patient escort.

David and I got engaged on Christmas Eve, 1975 when I was just 18 years old, and a freshman in Towson State College. Before our breakup, David and I had been together for 5 years, from age 14 to 19. In actuality, he was a father figure for me since my own father was so unavailable and emotionally detached from me. David was 7 years older than me, and very possessive. At times it seemed that his jealousy knew no boundaries. In the wake of the break-up, David, I found myself feeling very afraid, anxious and depressed because we had met and began our relationship when I was so very young and he had just graduated from college with a degree in zoology. He was such a big part of my life, a tremendous influence on me in my teen years. I had never had a broken heart from a relationship before. But I knew I had done the right thing in leaving him and - it was time for me to build a new life.

Though I was not allowed to date until I was 16, we first got together when he was 21 years old and had graduated from college, and I was just 14 years old. That would make him a pedophile by law. Our relationship certainly was not a 'normal' relationship due to the age difference.

Instead, it was one that should have never been. I suppose I was looking for a father figure as my own father had been so detached and unavailable. David was very controlling, protective and jealous, and I feared for my safety after I left him as I was never really sure what he was capable of doing to me if he found me. I was so afraid of him that I felt the need to transfer to another school that was outside of the Baltimore/Washington DC area.

On weekends, while a college freshman at Towson, I stayed with David and his parents in a small town near College Park, Maryland called Adelphi. As was frequently the case with most of my childhood friends and acquaintances, Howie somehow seemed to become fast friends with David' parents, without my ever introducing them. How and when I do not know. This was a regular pattern with my Dad and my friend's parents. Howie would inquire—actually, informally interview me-- about my school acquaintances, friends and dates, then locate and befriend them when I was not around, much to my surprise and chagrin. This unusual social pattern started in my early youth in Utica, New York and continued when we moved to Takoma Park, Maryland.

In fact, not sure why or how, but Howie often revealed to me that he knew more about my young schoolmates than even I did!

One night, while spending the weekend at David' parents' home on December 26th, 1975 just after getting an engagement ring from him for Christmas, I experienced my first grand mal seizure ever. The last thing I remember was drinking a soda David had given me. Subsequently, I was reportedly taken to the local hospital ER, and diagnosed with a seizure disorder. After the seizure, things became quite strained between us and he became sexually abusive. I called the wedding off, and left David just 2 months before the wedding after the abuse occurred. To this day, I will likely never know what happened to cause the seizure that fateful night; but I am eternally grateful that I did not marry that man.

Today, David is a disbarred pharmacist, incarcerated for Medicare/Medicaid fraud and OxyContin drug trafficking in Washington County, Maryland. Clearly, God had another plan for me that did not include him in my future! I consider this one more time that Jesus protected me in my youth, keeping me out of harm's way.

Not surprisingly, as I approached the 'age of freedom,' eighteen, I was depressed, overwhelmed and totally devastated by my daily life at home with mom, and weary of Howie's underworld antics. I truly felt that he had knowingly used me extensively in diversified ways, to build his Mob organization and to get what he wanted and thought he needed from his 'associates' and those he dis-enfranchised through his 'activities.' I was both confused, sad and angry, feeling used and abused, as I prepared to leave Takoma Park, Maryland and move to Baltimore for college.

Shortly after arriving at college in my freshman year, I sought counseling, but refused to believe I could be suffering from major depression or PTSD from the childhood trauma that I had endured, all the while repressing traumatic memories. However, careful to hardly ever speak about my childhood trauma with anyone, I put all of my energy into trying to forget my youth and focused on college life and becoming a registered nurse--something I had wanted to do since my mother became sick and went to the mental institution when I was a young child.

Howie's Big Exit

Well before cell phones, I remember getting a phone installed in my dorm room at college, specifically so I could call Howie, as it was my understanding that he still lived nearby in Middle River, Maryland. I had just seen him about a week before. Once my new phone was hooked up, I called him that Saturday afternoon to surprise him and to give him my new telephone number. Upon answering the phone, he asked me how I found him and told me never to call him again. Since he was secretive and had always been hesitant with me to provide his phone number, I found him through the telephone book. I was heart-broken, and cried for days.

Devastated, I wondered why he didn't want contact with me, though I suppose by that time, Howie and I had a love/hate relationship. I so wanted to have a better relationship with him as I remembered him in my very early youth when our family was still intact. But the reality was that that life had passed, and his double life with his associates had taken root in a really big way. I guess sometimes we all have illusions. Mine was that he loved me dearly, but the truth was that he and I were far past the point of a normal father-daughter relationship. In his utilitarian way, I guess that he no longer needed me to help him to unwittingly build his organization. Now I knew that the father-daughter relationship that I had treasured, even dreamed of as a young girl was no more, and as hard as it was, it was time I understood and accepted that harsh reality.

Then it happened. Just two days later, my mother called me to tell me Dad had reportedly "died" in a motel between Allentown and Harrisburg, PA where he was supposedly staying while on a business trip. My mother said that he had suffered a massive stroke and he had been found on the floor on Friday in his motel room some *3 days later after he 'died.'* That was a big surprise to me, impossible, in fact, as *I had just spoken with him on Saturday* afternoon after that time frame, and the dates did not match up! Besides, I thought…Three days—what motel wouldn't check and clean their rooms daily???

About 2 months after Howie's 'death,' my mother arranged for a Catholic memorial service for Howie, without his body present, to honor his life. He is now reportedly 'buried' at the Heavenly Gates Catholic Cemetery near Wheaton, Maryland, but I have no idea who transported his body from Allentown Harrisburg,

PA to Wheaton to the cemetery. I'm doubt it was my mother who arranged for it and paid for it, since she had no financial resources to do so. Howie had no head stone for about two years due to lack of finances in our family. However, one day, one just appeared.

It is noteworthy, that since Howie "passed," I have seen him in person three times since Sept 10th, 1975. The first was in Baltimore City, the most recent time was circa 2006 also in Baltimore City, and once in Las Vegas, NV when I was giving a talk there in 2000. Given his ilk, and the double life that Howie led with the Mob before he "passed," his unsavory associates, and his lawless 'activities,' perhaps I should not be surprised that it appears that he faked his own death. I can only guess why he did it, but I will likely never know for sure.

Fast Forward

About 40 years later, through online research, I learned that the summer Howie reportedly 'died' two of his close New York/New Jersey Mob associates, our former neighbor John Roselli/ aka Filippo Sacco [August 9th, 1975] and his longtime associate Sam Giancana [June 19th, 1975] were both murdered just before Howie's reported death. and Filippo Sacco, one of our incarcerated neighbors in Utica, NY. Another one of Howie's business associates, Union Boss Jimmy Hoffa, whom he talked about often, went missing July 30th, 1975, just 5 weeks before Howie's 'Big Exit.' In retrospect, it is highly possible that Howie's World had become so dangerous that he had to disappear on September 10th, 1975 when the heat was on. Perhaps he thought he was next.

If Howie were alive today, as of this writing, which is extremely doubtful, he would be 93 years old. My last Howie citing was about 10 years ago when he would have been around 83 years old. As for Howie's likely geographical location, I have no idea. However, in as much as no one lives forever, old age has probably taken its toll and it is highly <u>unlikely</u> Howie is still alive. Only God knows where he would be if he were still alive.

Repeatedly encountering Howie's local associates, together with subsequent PTSD flashbacks and nightmares, propelled me to write about my early family life with Howie and Gina. At first it was quite difficult and extremely distressing, then became much less so, as I slowly, eventually, began remembering events, and pieces of the puzzle of my life started to come together and make sense over time.

HOWIE, CHARLIE AND THE FIRST "APALACHIN" MEETING

One day I was talking with a man I had known for about 10 years named Charlie. Charlie was a gruff sort, an Italian American with a quick wit and a swaggering boldness about him. He talked incessantly about his 'compadres,' his 'Gumbas,' and their tough guy antics, often to my chagrin. I never knew what he would say next, but one day he apparently had something to tell me:

"*Hey Adele! I **know** your father!*" he said with a smile.

"*My father? How do you know my father?*" I asked trying to act like it was no big deal, but it was a very big deal, as it was I still believed that my father had reportedly "died" years prior to the conversation.

"*He was at the first Apalachin meeting.*"

"*How do YOU know?*" I asked with all the forced indignation I could muster.

"*Because it was at my house in Apalachin, New York!*"

I'm not sure what I said after that, but I knew what he was telling me was important in understanding my father's world. Many, many years later, I looked up the First Apalachin Meeting on the internet, and was shocked by what I learned. The First Apalachin was an historic event in November 1957 of the American Mafia. It was the reportedly the first and largest American underworld organizational meeting of the American Mafia including all the crime families of New York/New Jersey with over 100 mobsters present! I was crestfallen and baffled.

How in the world did Charlie possibly know my father in the present tense since he had reportedly died in September 1975? If what he was saying was true, it meant that Howie was still alive and had participated in this meeting when I was just 6 months old! With Dad's bent towards lawlessness, and his early background living in the Bronx, it all seemed to make sense and was also even more validation of *'Birds of a Feather Flock Together.'* For me, this single piece of information served as the biggest red flag of all for the other déjà vu experiences and nuances I had lived through. From that point forward, I felt like I had a new and most uncomfortable understanding about Howie and his world. However, somehow still wanting to think the best of Dad, I buried the memory until it resurfaced in later years. Actually, this memory re-emergedwhen I first learned about "Uncle Meyer" Lansky from the TV documentary about the New York/New Jersey crime families, as the show had talked about the First Apalachin meeting.

Clearly, dealing with the unknown is hard—harder in fact—than facing cold truth. Eventually, I became able to find purpose in knowing about Howie's World--praying for him and his associates who were involved in various aspects of his activities, and it gave me great relief to do so. Why? Because I believe every soul can repent and turn to God, regardless of past "activities."

In fact, in the Catholic tradition, I continue to pray for them by name and my prayers for them includes the **Divine Mercy Prayer:**

"Oh my Jesus, forgive us our sins, save us from the fires of Hell, and lead all souls to Heaven, especially those in most need of Thy mercy."

What I did not fully realize when I first started writing, was that though the writing process was very, very challenging for me, it helped me heal. I was able to reframe my childhood experience with the power of God's grace, and the help of my therapist and psychiatrist, and move on unencumbered. As time went on, with each writing session, I felt lighter, and freer inside; less burdened, less anxious, less stressed, and more comfortable in my own skin than ever before.

Today, by the grace of God, I am able to pray specifically for those who hurt me most by name, and especially for those who turned their heads to the abuse I endured. I am able to pray for my own healing, in body, mind and spirit, as well. Reliving and reprocessing the trauma of my youth is one of the hardest things I have ever done in my life—but necessary for my physical and mental health. It is clearly, also one of the most beneficial things I have done for myself.

Yes, I wrote what came day and night; and as I did so, clarity came, with each writing, and, more and more. I realized that I had for years felt misplaced shame and guilt relating to my childhood experience and family, especially with Howie.

Today, I walk in the sublime confidence that my prayers are being answered and that I am deeply loved by God, my *Heavenly Father*. As I have grown in my ability to forgive the unforgivable, I have made great strides in healing in mind, body and spirit, and that confidence has allowed me to grow spiritually like never before. Today I have a deep, abiding peace, and joy to share with others. I feel lighter and more carefree as I have become less burdened, and I can't wait to see the personal healing that is ahead and what Jesus will do next in my life!

> *Whatever you were yesterday, or even this morning, has passed. Today, through God's sublime gifts of the power of forgiveness, grace and salvation, You are a New Creation, in Jesus Christ!*
>
> Adele M. Gill

Are you ready to lay down your heavy burden, your angst, your worry, your frustration, your un-forgiveness and brokenness to begin a new, hope-filled life in Jesus right now, today, my friend?

If so, the Bible tells us, *"Go in peace."* Perhaps it may be a blessed good time to let it go. Seek the Lord, and you will surely find Him. Prepare to embrace your God-given purpose and bask in the sun as you feel the warmth of His unconditional love. Have you ever felt as if God has forgotten you and does not answer your prayers? Of course you have! But sometimes it helps if you lean in, and take a closer look and listen quietly to what God has in store for you. He's always up to something good on your behalf!

Now I understand that I never have been, and never will be, given more than I can endure, as God and his elect are watching over me, and you, day and night, 24/7. He has given me exactly what I needed in EVERY circumstance, in perfect time, as His grace is sufficient. For Our Dear Lord is kind & merciful. Like any truly Good Father, he stands in wait to provide for our every need, and is ever-present to those who seek Him in earnest.

God promises to fill all our needs, and is ever faithful to be sure we have what we need in good measure, especially when we ask in the name of Jesus! Go ahead and ask for what you need in prayer in the most specific way, and see how He fulfills His promise to provide abundantly for each of us. For I have found that when you are very specific with God in prayer, He will be specific with you when answering your prayers!

I simply cannot imagine this journey I have traveled, this life I have lived, without the love and the Light of Jesus Christ, *the greatest hope and love I have ever known.* Yes, some difficult things that happened in my youth have bubbled up over the years, but the most painful, traumatic events and things endured have been much slower to come to the foreground. Through therapy, much prayer, and many sleepless nights, my childhood-lost has re-emerged in my conscious brain, and though difficult to deal with at times, I am forever and eternally grateful for the opportunity to *heal from the inside out, in mind, body and spirit.*

Certainly no life is all pain and struggle, as we all have joy and blessings that resonate, even from within the depths of the darkest times in our lives. Yet, for some, the agony of living with an unspeakable childhood trauma, with innocence lost early on, can be an enduring source of discontentment in life, emotional upheaval, medical issues, and even for some, seething, unresolved anger and bitterness even into old age.

If that sounds all too familiar, perhaps this book was written for you. It is my expressed hope that by sharing some of my own childhood experiences through this book, that I will be able to help many others who live with untreated childhood trauma and subsequently, similar emotional or mental health issues, chronic neurological and/or autoimmune infirmity, to begin the healing process.

May Our Dear Lord wrap His loving arms around you, help remove any and all embedded thorn(s) that remain from any childhood trauma you have experienced, and heal you fully in mind, body and soul, as well.

Amen!

CHOOSING TO LIVE IN TODAY

"Therefore, do not worry about tomorrow, for tomorrow will worry about itself. Each day has enough trouble of its own."

Matthew 6:34

If you need to look at the past for healing of mind and body, due to untreated childhood trauma, remember this—*the past is a place to visit, not to dwell*. Look back too long, and you may risk missing all that is unfolding before you today. You may even literally run into obstacles and things that could easily have been avoided. I now believe it is important to face situations as they occur, process them the best way you can, and pray about everything.

In my case, it was imperative that I heal from untreated childhood trauma to ease the depression and infirmity that developed in my early adult life. Today, understanding *The Mind-Body-Faith Phenomenon©*, I have come to the realization that I am forced to recognize, despite my own reservations, that my present, particularly my health, is largely controlled by untreated childhood trauma. Because of this reality, I have to guard against fatigue, infection, and stress that can trip my neuro-immune system causing an exacerbation of the myasthenia-like syndrome, as well as, monitor angst, depression, and despair. Most of all, I need to recognize that Jesus is and has been with me through it all.

When I am living in the past, I can only see the pain and torment of my growing up years, and it is easy to fall into depression and angst, as sometimes my soul becomes turbulent, devoid of peace, and even angry for what was, and how my untreated childhood trauma seems to control the present through my health.

Yet through the eyes of faith, everything looks different. When I take a closer look at my upbringing, I see how God prepared me for living with the infirmity I now live with. Yes, I now believe I will be healed one day as I am on the 'miracle installment plan." I'm not sure how, but by the grace of God, I am confident that I will be infirmity-free one day. The depression has for the most part, been healed with therapy and medication, and I am reclaiming my life as I tell my story and break the silence of my youth. Having put my childhood to rest, I am at peace and experience much joy in my life as I am able to live in the here and now far more easily.

Though every day is clearly a new adventure filled with surprises, I am able to say now that my childhood and mind-body conditions no longer define me. It just is what it is, and I live one day at a time in gratitude to Jesus for all the blessings he has bestowed on me and my loved ones.

Yes, I still have unwelcome childhood memories bubble up; but they no longer overwhelm me.

In fact, since I have been writing these memories down, I am freer than ever to live a happy life, to love those that God has put in my life, and to experience joy, even in adversity. For when I live in the present, I am much more capable of living a peaceful, joy-filled, productive life, taking the time to appreciate myself and others, and stopping to smell the flowers along the way.

Living in the here and now, I have time and energy to do my best, and pray for those I cherish, and those I do not love as I should in my life.

I am able to be available for my family and those in need of support, and encouragement, able to reach out to the poor, the elderly, and the infirm as Christ asks us to do. In fact, having had the childhood and life experiences I have had has prepared me to be more compassionate to others, more forgiving, more empathetic. I know what it is like to be hungry, poor, rejected, abandoned and abused. I know how these things can produce a hurting soul. Conversely, I understand the long road back from these places of the heart to living a full live. In essence, I know well what it means to be broken, really broken, seemingly beyond repair, and what it takes to find your way to higher ground.

Take a closer look at how you are living your life this day. Are you riddled with anguish for what could have been, what has been lost, or taken from you, prematurely, in your youth, mid-life or later years?

Look too far ahead of you, and through the lapse of time, you risk missing the day you are commissioned to live in the here and now. Perhaps it is a good time to discover that your past is just is what it is—recognizing that it is beyond your control. However, understand that you can learn from your past experiences and mistakes, *choose to live in the present,* and plan for a better future for you and your family.

Do you spend much of your time and energy in the future fighting the demons of fear, dread, sadness, or loneliness over what is to come? If so, now is the time to stop and take stock... Take a deep breath, and look at all the blessings that surround you this day. If you need to, start a daily gratitude list-one that includes who and what is treasured in your life, what is most important to you in the here and now.

Soon you will begin to trust that yesterday and tomorrow really will take care of themselves. For when we let go of the burdens of yesterday, which have passed, and tomorrow, which will come despite our anguish, we are more able to embrace the rich, new blessings that The Lord has for us with each new sunrise, each new day. Yes, it is difficult, if not impossible for many to rejoice when you are steeped in troubles and adversity. However, I find that when I fully focus on Jesus, in gratitude for all my blessings, I am lifted in a way like no other. For me, just repeating the name Jesus is enough to cast out fear and angst and get me back on track.

Lift up your heart and head today... Pray to be free in Jesus! Soon you will see your health improve in body, mind and spirit, leaving you prepared to meet each day with peace, serenity, and joy--God's great gifts for hope-filled souls that place their trust in Him!

Dad, on the other hand presented as 'Fun-time Charlie,' always ready for an adventure. When he would pick us up on his visitation weekends, we never knew what adventure was ahead for us, where he would take us, or what we would be doing which only heightened the excitement. He introduced us to so many unusual experiences that children were not often allowed to do. In my mind, each visit was separate unto itself, and Howie was very careful never to help me connect the dots as to the locations where we went, the people he exposed me to, and the experiences we had. But there was one thing for sure. Each visit ended with what became a most predictable admonition from my father, *'Don't tell your mother or anyone about this.'*

There was also an implied threat that if we told Mom, she would not let us be with him on visitation days. When we lived in Utica, Howie took us summer after summer time and again to 'Tony's Camp' on Hinckley Lake in Upstate New York. It was an adult-only camp with a large sign posted: *"NO CHILDREN ALLOWED."* Per my observations, it was a swinger's club on a lake where people 'shared' partners. For some reason I am fully unaware of, we three kids were allowed there. *"Just don't tell..."* Tony was actually the court appointed, assigned social worker for my mom and us kids after their divorce. Dad definitely had a way of quickly gaining allegiance from people he met in the most unusual of ways from all walks of life, and Tony at Camp Hinckley was one shining example.

Shortly before Howie's his "Big Exit," he had a meeting and asked us to drop him off and pick him up in an hour and a half at a Greek Restaurant in Highlandtown/Baltimore, Maryland. When we went to pick him up, he was meeting with a young Saudi man who was in full Middle Eastern dress with head wrap, named Abdullah Shaikh Mohammed. I asked him how to spell his name, and he did so with great arrogance, clarifying that it was spelled "Shaikh," not "Sheikh." I asked briefly about the weather in Saudi Arabia. *"It's very hot in Saudi Arabia. You'll get used to it!"* he said, to my dismay. He seemed to have a wonderful command of the English language. Yet his words echoed in my mind for many years wondering what he meant. With that said, I reassured him I had no plans of ever going there, though what he said to me made me wonder what their meeting was about. When we returned home after the weekend, Howie had his usual admonition: *"Don't tell anyone,"* and I didn't, for many years-- who would believe me anyway?

By the grace of God, through PTSD flashbacks, nightmares and much therapy, I have been able to successfully look back, and reframe my traumatic childhood with the help of a wonderful psychiatrist and therapist team who worked together to guide me through the therapy process, and to heal. After decades of angst, I wrote about my youth with the Lord at my side, it seemed to lift the heavy burdens of my heart and soul, one event at a time, off of my shoulders more and more. Each new childhood memory was yet another opportunity to debride the shrapnel and heal the wounds that had had festered and controlled my well-being.

If I had been capable of fully understanding the gravity of many of the events and experiences from my childhood as they occurred to me, I likely would have given up in fear, angst and despair at an early age. But the Lord is kind and merciful, gently leading us in His perfect timing and way. Protector, Comforter, Healer, Almighty Savior…I can hardly count all the times there were close calls and Jesus came to my aid in the most practical ways!

Unlike computer technology, there is no replay, forward, delete, or rewind in this life. We have been blest with just one day at a time. Who could possibly live in the past, present, and the future at the same time and still embrace the blessings presented by each and every new day? We would crumble under the pressure. I know this because I tried. We only really have today, memories of yesteryear, and the hope of tomorrow; yet, due to our humanness, we are only able to fully live and process one day at a time. For each day is a blessed time capsule unto itself.

Remembering Childhood Trauma

There is a certain readiness that occurs with many people that leads them to be able to talk about and deal with untreated traumatic childhood memories as they bubble up. For most, there comes a time when they must face, and deal with, traumatic events that have occurred in their lives so they can heal and move on to embrace the healing that awaits them. Nowhere is that more prevalent and true than with adult survivors of children of trauma. I tried my best to just get on with living, but by the age of 49, I could no longer emotionally avoid the elephant in the room. I had hit the proverbial wall of my childhood, and subsequently adult realities.

Eventually, I was flooded day and night with old memories of people, faces, names, places, and the like, from Gina and Howie's worlds, I found myself writing it all down, journaling for the purposes of clarity and deep healing. In truth, I did not know what else to do with the memories as they invaded my day time serenity, my senses, my very peace of mind, and even my sleep at night time. So I continued to write down the details and memories that came upon me.

To my surprise, however, through the tumult and torment, I eventually grew so that I no longer needed anyone to tell me where I had been, what had occurred in my family in my youth, and in my turbulent, traumatic childhood, as the missing pieces of my life puzzle entered my conscious mind. Finally, I was able to connect the dots! Gratefully, by the grace of God, over time, my memory has been restored, much forgiveness has taken place, and I am at peace once again as I pray often and fervently for those I have known in my life in most need of God's mercy, especially the Five Families of New York.

Difficult as it all was, no longer did a code of silence about life events rule my conscious and subconscious mind, as I was able to write, discuss in therapy, and name and claim whathappened. Through therapy, eventually, the uncomfortable feelings from the recollections of past memories began to fade, and they were replaced with a sense of calm as the memories simply became just part of the fabric of my daily life. Through quiet prayer and much psychotherapy, I have been fully able to name, claim and reframe my personal childhood trauma in a positive light to restore and reflect what I have always known in my heart:

"All things work for good for those who love God."

Romans 8:28

There are many things that can help traumatic memories resurface. Going to certain places, dreams, PTSD nightmares, flashbacks, seeing certain people, experiencing certain familiar feelings, smelling certain smells, writing, and of course, therapy, are just a few ways that traumatic childhood memories can be brought to the foreground from years gone by. These events and sensations may trip long forgotten memories, allowing them to resurface to be dealt with effectively.

So what happens when you are an adult and become flooded with traumatic childhood memories through dreams, PTSD nightmares, flashbacks and the like? In my case, I realized that it must be time to deal with the past events or the memories would not be bubbling up. In my mind, once I got my bearings, I decided that it was God's perfect timing for healing inside and out. In the beginning while recalling these experiences, I fell three times into a downhill spiraling depression and felt despair as I remembered the early trauma in my life. In fact, flooded with memories, I was completely overwhelmed by, and adverse to, even the thought of reliving my traumatic childhood. Though I often had the same traumatic dreams and flashbacks 2-3 times, I tried three different times over a period of a year and a half to write down what came to me to no avail. However, finally, with the fourth try, I began to write out what came to me in corroborative memories, PTSD flashbacks and nightmares, and I was finally successful in beginning to be able to wade through the sadness and angst. It felt like a fever breaking. Make no mistake about it, it was hard to do--really hard.

What freedom it was once I realized that these memories had

bubbled up for a reason. With Jesus at my side, it was time to deal with what happened in my childhood as it was so painful, since the memories had been repressed for decades. I realized that it was time to heal old hurts of my traumatic youth by gently reopening the wounds, removing the thorns and shrapnel, and healing the old wounds.

No longer was I bound by the code of silence of my family and those that were self-imposed. No longer could I allow myself to be hurt by glimpses and visions of the haunting events that happened many decades ago. No more could I pretend that nothing happened out of the ordinary in my youth. I felt empowered to talk about it, but soon realized that the intensity of my childhood trauma was not necessarily something that other people were ready to hear—Certainly not my husband, my friends, my priests, not my siblings--only my therapist and psychiatrist were up to hearing what had transpired in my early family life. So I wrote and wrote, and prayed and prayed, and wrote some more, and it was the best therapy ever!

For decades these memories have been 'bubbling up' a little at a time, but in recent years, it has been more like a volcanic eruption. At first, I was deeply distressed by even the thought of reliving where I had been. Then I realized that God was in control here, and He would not give me more than I could handle more than He and I could handle together. The relief I experienced from that thinking point forward was not only inspiring, but very healing, and blest!

Not really knowing what to do as the memories came up with great detail, I began writing them down exactly as they came to me with raw emotion. I soon noticed that what came in dreams and nightmares was corroborated by what came through PTSD flashbacks and vice versa. In fact, these experiences were also corroborated by the puzzle pieces I already held in my heart and mind. In turn, I shared with my therapist, who was very helpful in showing me how to get a healthy perspective, how to reframe my memories, put them in their place, and put them to rest for good. *And, with time, what a relief it was!*

Unable to live comfortably in the harshness of the present day, while struggling to look to the future, I looked ahead, often with forced optimism, as my childhood mantra in middle school and high school became, *"This, too, shall pass!"* It has been said that "God will make a way, when there seems to be no way." And I KNOW He made a way for me to heal and grow through this 'dark night of the soul' experience.

It is doubtful that I would be writing this book if not for having gone through these childhood experiences. Emotionally and spiritually, I am far stronger now than I have ever been in my life, in my faith, in my relationships, and happy to give credit where credit is due. For Jesus Christ has always been with me, has never left my side through it all, and I am ever so grateful. Today, my past, present, and future belong to Him, and I feel as though my life is blest!

Yes, revisiting, naming and claiming my traumatic childhood was difficult, but it brought me closer to God in all His glory, and was the necessary path to healing old emotional wounds. In stark comparison to my parents, I have come to truly embrace Jesus as my Savior, not only in the 'church' sense, but in the most practical ways imaginable, as I am ever thankful for His steadfast love and care for me.

My relationship with Howie, which damaged my ability to trust people, especially, has led me to seek Jesus with all my heart. As a result, I realize that Jesus' love for me is infinitely more powerful than my darkest days with Howie and Gina. I am now able to rise above the fray, and reach for my Savior's hand, no longer being dragged down by hatred and unforgiveness for Howie, his world, and his 'associates.' I finally understand that God decided long before I was born what family I would be in, and my parents were part of His selection for me in my life.

Through my Mom, I learned much about endurance and love; through Howie, I learned just how good God really is, and how unconditional His Love is for all of us. In as much as God is the very definition of love, Howie's world class antics and 'activities' actually pale in comparison with the Lord's grace, kindness and goodness. Even as Howie went about trying to discredit God publicly at the Unitarian Universalist Society, the Lord was lifting me up in holy boldness, discernment and integrity to rise above his sordid ways. In the end, we are all accountable for what we do and say, and Howie will have to answer for himself.

Most of all, now, I am now able to pray for Howie and his comrades, like never with focus like never before. I pray often, and have for years prayed for the 5 families of New York, their extended 'families,' and for Howie's associates. In my mind, in my way of thinking, I do not need to forget what transpired that sent me reeling in my youth and into adulthood. Rather, now, I am certain that it is far more important to be able to pray fervently for those who hurt me than to struggle with the ongoing effects of a lack unforgiveness.

I learned at an early age, and in a very personal way, that God is Almighty, kind and merciful, and His love and care are beyond comparison. I learned that Jesus is ever present to each of us, even and especially providing practical help in times of trouble, and, unlike others in my life, that He would never, ever hurt me or leave me. That Jesus went before His flock always to pave the way, and behind every sheep to protect them.

Through prayer and therapy, my memory regarding the many traumatic childhood events in my childhood has slowly returned and I am now more in awe of Jesus and His perfect timing more than ever before. Although it is hard to believe, my mother's mental illness and subsequent abject cruelty, and Howie's neglect, abuse, and illegal 'activities' seem to pale in contrast to the great love, comfort and protection that flows from Jesus!

Having been in harm's way plenty in my youth, especially with Howie and David, I marvel at how Jesus preserved me as His own! I am blown away by His unconditional love!!! I can hardly find the words to express my gratitude to the Lord for all the blessings I received throughout my childhood—even, and especially, through all the trauma.

Jesus is and was my Great Protector, Gentle Comforter and Consoler, my Almighty Counselor and Guide, the Lover of My Soul. He was my bright light in the dark tunnel of oppression in my youth; my Strength in weakness, and my Joy in captivity while living with my mother. Words cannot express my gratitude for how Jesus preserved me and my siblings through it all. Yes, we all have our scars, yet my heart leaps when I think of how Jesus provided for me all that I needed through times of neglect and abuse of every kind. I will never forget how Jesus protected me with His right arm just as the Bible tells us, never letting anyone snatch me from His far-reaching care.

However, this much I do know; all I want to do is serve God with all my body, strength, mind, and soul in this life, and be with Him for eternity in the next! Living a faith-filled life has its own challenges, as it is no guarantee that you will not experience the fullness of human life.

Physical infirmity, disability, stress, poverty, strained relationships, etc…may easily encroach on one's ability to stay focused on God. However, *with God, all things are possible.* It is possible and important to experience peace and joy *despite* adversity; as Jesus helps carry our burdens and gives us the strength to press on, and do the best we can with each and every day in every circumstance. For when we focus on God's strength, healing and unmerited grace to help us along, we are much better able to face whatever befalls us in this life.

SILVER LINING

As an adult, I am in awe of the saving power of unconditional love, hope, grace, and trust in Jesus Christ. Little did I know in my youth that His saving power would benefit generations in my family once I could hand my life and family over to Jesus. And I mean everything--all of the pain, the torment, the abuse, the evil that surrounded me, all of it handed over trustingly to Jesus to sort out, to sustain me, to provide for my every need and that of my husband and our children.

Yes, my youth was, by all accounts, harrowing, and riddled with mayhem, chaos, abuse, and danger. Yet, I am here to tell you that it was by the grace of God that I survived living with both my parents. Despite having seen and lived with gut-wrenching poverty, my mother's acute and chronic mental illness, and Dad's double life and propensity for lawlessness with the Mob, I came to appreciate God and to grow in deep faith in my youth. I had to turn to Jesus, as there was nowhere else to turn.

In my own way, in my youth, I guess I often staved off relationships in an effort to protect myself and the home life I lived from being known, by containing school friendships to school hours. The fact that I was grounded much of the time from middle school to high school, unable to go out with friends or even talk with them on the phone after school and on weekends, only increased the isolation I felt and lived.

Early on, in middle school, I obtained a copy of the Holy Bible and kept it under my bed to read when in forced isolation, or what I called 'Mom's lockdown.' According to my mother, I was not allowed to read the Bible while I lived in her home, as it was considered contraband. She believed that only a Catholic priest had the discernment to read the Holy Bible. Quite honestly, praying and reading the Bible kept me sane while dealing with my mother. I especially loved reading the praise-filled Book of Psalms and the four synoptic Gospels: Matthew, Luke, Mark and John. The Beatitudes/Sermon on the Mount, *"Blessed are the poor in spirit, theirs is the Kingdom of God"* gave me great comfort in my youth. I also loved reading the Psalms as they were brimming with hope for the poor, the vulnerable, the oppressed, and the hurting. And as I read them, I became more able to pray fervently for Gina and Howie, and especially his associates, something I do to this day in a more specific way now that I have so many more pieces of the puzzle to Howie's World etched in my heart and mind. I especially pray fervently now for the "5 families of New York, naming each associate I can remember, and their "extended families," as well as all of Howie's associates involved in violence, racketeering, trafficking, drugs, gambling, the unions, the markets, extortion, graft, and 'the adult entertainment industry.' I also pray for those who he unwittingly used in the pursuit of his illicit activities.

Before coming to know Jesus as my personal Savior, Healer, Comforter, and Friend, I especially leaned a lot on Blessed Mother for strength and courage to get through the day. My mother used to have an iconic painting of Mary and baby Jesus on the wall in her bedroom. So many times, during her times of cruel psychosis, I would catch a glimpse out of the corner of my eye of the picture of Blessed Mother Mary lovingly holding Jesus, and it would help me to stay focused on my faith rather than her wrath. This practice alone was enough to keep me going in my youth with a resilient spirit and blessed holy boldness.

In a way, that picture represented the mother I never had. So gentle, kind, and loving, Mary was, for me, the loving mother I had always wanted, and I considered God to be my Father. I never really had a mother to turn to and share my life with as it was unfolding. My early life was an endurance test that beckoned me to rise above my family circumstances, to dig deep for what was good and right and true, to continually deal with hunger, torment and poverty, and to hold fast onto my faith like driftwood in a turbulent, rushing river bed flowing down stream.

As the years passed, my allegiance to Mary changed, as I realized that Jesus Himself was my personal Savior. To this day, I turn to Him for my every need, great and small. Some people say that we should only pray to Jesus for big things. I totally disagree. Rather, I believe that He wants us to pray for the little things too, and to be the center of our lives. And for me, He is and has been exactly that for years!

In all the mayhem, I learned at an early age to look for silver linings in every circumstance, every adversity, so much so, that my parents called me 'Bright Eyes.' Though I was truly limited in being able to console or comfort my mother as she often cycled through paranoid delusions, cruel psychotic rants and weeping bitterly while praying out loud day and night for God to 'take her,' I tried my best to be as supportive as possible, but to stay out of her way out of self-preservation.

CHAPTER 5:
Uncharted Waters: The College Years

*"So do not fear, I am with you;
do not be dismayed, for I am your God.
I will strengthen you and help you;
I will uphold you with my righteous right hand."*

Isaiah 41:10

LIVING ON THE EDGE

I would love to be able to say that I lived through my traumatic childhood and came out un-scathed, but that is simply not so. In fact, it is far from the truth.

At the age of 18, between trying to cope with what I believed to be the "passing" of my father, keeping my toxic mother, and her ranting psychoses at bay, being diagnosed with epilepsy the year before, and the break-up with my fiancé, David, I felt totally overwhelmed by life at-large.

After the break-up with David in June of 1976, when I was 18, I transferred from State College for my second year of pre-nursing, to Frostburg State College, and lived with my sister there for the summer to mend my broken heart. Initially, when I got to Frostburg, I lived off campus with my sister and her roommates in the apartment upstairs for the summer. Since my sister had just graduated, she moved out at the end of the summer and I arranged to move into a newly renovated rental house across the street. I did not tell David the address of where I was going to live, as I was in fear that he would try to find me. My fears were well grounded – I later learned that he had come to Frostburg on two separate occasions to look for me.

One evening while at college, I went out for a while and came back to find one of my roommate's very upset. She said that several people had burst into our house and our room looking for me. They turned over chairs and tables in the kitchen, destroyed property, and yelled my name through the house. They even stole my only winter coat that was in the hallway on a rack. My roommate said she and her boyfriend were so frightened that they hid under her bed waiting for the men to leave, and were unable to describe them. By the grace of God, no one found them hiding under the bed. It is highly likely that that it was David looking for me, as I can't imagine who else it would have been.

When I heard what happened, I became afraid that whoever it was would return, but they never did. We lived in an old, renovated house, with a beautiful winding staircase, several fireplaces, and tall ceilings with clap-board shutters. The house had been the old Republican Club, and though renovated, still had the original long bar and bar stools in the kitchen. The house was like something out of a movie. There were 6 women who lived there together. At one time it had been an old, historic Civil War house, and though I never ventured down into the basement, the rumor was that it that it connected to the basements of other local homes that were part of the Civil War "Underground Railroad."

In a way, I felt great freedom in Frostburg being away from home. David had become very controlling, jealous, and abusive. I was also concerned for my safety as I prayed he wouldn't find me. Though I had dreamed of the wonderful freedom I would have when I left home, I was quite unprepared for what my newly found freedom really meant, and began frequenting the local bar, 'The

Reef,' with friends several times a week. I also attended many mixers and frat parties with friends in an effort to numb the emotional pain of all that had transpired with David and my traumatic youth, I turned to alcohol to self-medicate as the emotional pain was relentless.

Alcohol was easily accessible and seemed to be an integral part of college life. Essentially, while in college, I went through a very difficult 2 year period where I stepped away from my family, and David, out of the need for self-preservation. Moreover, I also walked away from Jesus for the first time in my life. During this period, I had briefly seen a counselor who told me my mother was toxic for me. This gave me 'permission' of sorts to step back, and take care of myself emotionally. I continued to call my mother occasionally out of respect for her being my mother, but I visited very infrequently to avoid the mental abuse and the subsequent searing pain.

I loved my mother, but I did not like the way she treated me at all. I always felt like I wasn't good enough by her standards, that I was a disappointment to her. But the truth was bigger than that-as my mother repeatedly told me that she held me responsible for the breakup of her marriage to my father. These feelings dated back to when she was pregnant with me and started having epileptic seizures. She always said that Howie didn't want me, or her after she was diagnosed, and he wanted her to abort me. I cared deeply for my mother, despite the way she treated me, but I think it is fair to say I hated her cruelty.

The times when I did call home, my mother was so mentally abusive, that I became afraid of her, and I cried after each contact. Additionally, I would have upsetting nightmares about our tumultuous relationship for days, even weeks after. After just one phone call, I would be clinically depressed, and could feel my self-esteem withering, as contact with her left me feeling unloving, and unloved. Her words haunted me:

"You'll never be anything..."
"You'll never become a nurse..."
"I'm sorry you were ever born..."
"I should have aborted you like your Dad wanted me to."
"You're the reason I am divorced."

Her words of dire criticism, malice and hatred flooded my soul and echoed in my mind for days, even weeks. After she was done castigating me, I could hardly focus or function. Yet she always proclaimed that she was the innocent victim in our relationship and she was going to have a heart attack and die because of my calls, or because I did not visit at regular intervals. Her approach to life and our relationship was not unlike Fred Sanford on the Sanford and Sons Show. In that show, Fred Sanford was always threatening to have a heart attack and die when faced with social challenges. Despite these claims that started when she was in her 50's, Mom lived to the ripe age of 92, outliving both her siblings!

Though my siblings seemed to more easily handle her psychoses, her phone calls to me were riddled with torment, anger, paranoid delusions and untrue malicious accusations that cut me like a knife. The sad truth was, her phone calls left me speechless and in despair. Usually, I just wept quietly after she had her psychotic phone rants, while admonishing myself for calling her or answering the phone in the first place. I always hoped and dreamed that I could one day 'fix' my mother's mental and physical health. This goal probably led me to wanting to be a nurse from the young age of four.

Once I left home, I knew there was no returning there, as her cruelty had reached its pinnacle, and I could no longer subject myself to her abuse. Long before cell phones, she would regularly call me on our community house phone only to hang up, and then call back a few minutes later.

Sometimes she would immediately call me back 20 times or more for round two saying, *"I'm going to die and it will be all your fault!"* and *"You know I am not supposed to get upset!"* Long before caller ID, I soon learned that I had to fight the temptation to answer the phone, or to call her, as her mean-spirited cruelty made it hard for me to study, have relationships, and function at all.

After any contact with Mom, I felt deflated, with nowhere to turn to share either my feelings of worthlessness or the excitement of college life. There was no mom to share my good grades with; no mom to ask for advice, or to encourage me along in my relationships and studies. I dreaded her calls and often did not answer the phone out of self-preservation. I vowed if I ever had children, I would love them dearly, encourage them along, and work hard to help them build their self-esteem. My self-worth was diminished and depleted by this woman I called Mom, whose hatred and malice seemed to lower my self-esteem with each contact.

Fast Forward

Today, I understand that my mother suffered dearly with mental illness for most of her adult life.

Her life was extremely hard, and my father left her when she needed him most. She always reverted to telling me he left her because of her being diagnosed with epilepsy while pregnant with me. But that was certainly not my fault as I wasn't even born yet.

Amongst her 3 children, I was the focus of her anger, angst and rages. Mostly, I think I reminded her of herself in her youth as I was sassy and so full of life. Also, we both had epilepsy, I look themost like her of her three children, and we both lived with depression. Perhaps she saw her own reflection in me and it startled her.

THE REEF

In the fall of 1976, when I was 19, while at the local pub called, *The Reef*, someone apparently put some sort of date rape drug in my beer, likely rufinol or ecstacy. That night, I was gang raped after coming home from the bar to the house where I lived on Main Street. Just prior to being drugged, I was with one of my roommates, and some of her visiting friends, including two young men named 'Mickey' and 'Bill.' They supposedly were there with a visiting football team from another school in the town where one of my roommate's lived.

Though I have little, if any memory of what happened, which in and of itself is very telling, I reportedly passed out at the bar after drinking about half of a beer, and woke up briefly as I heard my friend say, *"Take her home boys!"* They carried me home, which was about a block away.

I remember waking up briefly in my apartment during the rape and seeing 5 to 7 strangers in my room and bright lights. The next morning I woke up and *soon realized what had happened.* I felt groggy and defiled, so violated, so alone, but had no conscious recollection whatsoever of what had happened to me! After that, my life came to a screeching halt in every way, physically, academically, socially, mentally, emotionally, and spiritually.

I considered withdrawing from school, but wondered, 'where would I go?' and 'what would I do?' It was sheer will and faith in Jesus Christ that kept me going after what had happened. Yet pressing questions flooded my mind faster than I could process them. Was I simply in the wrong place at the wrong time, or was it something more premeditated, I wondered. One of my roommate's father and Howie were both engineers and long-time associates. Could the rape have happened at the hands of someone I knew, or perhaps even someone who knew my ex-fiancé, David, or someone else from 'Howie's World???' I will likely never know. The only thing I was sure about was that the pain of what had happened that fateful night rocked me and my world to my core, even to my weary soul.

It did not take long for me to finally realize that I needed Jesus back in my life. I needed to feel His arms around me once again, and to reach out for His hand with the trust of a young child. I needed His healing touch, and to be comforted. Lord, I needed Jesus back in my life as I felt very, vulnerable, alone and fragile. It was a desolate time in my life, filled with angst and despair, much like walking over a tight rope without a safety net. In hindsight, I have learned through Scripture that it is important to note that when suffering takes you to the brink, it often produces patience and perseverance, and is the reason for undergirding resilience, something God had instilled in me from my youth. I had to believe that God really doesn't give us more than we can handle. For me, resilience and compassion came from turning to God in prayer and continuing to press on in faith, even when confronted with overwhelming, heinous life events.

With ample, overwhelming burdens and plenty of emotional baggage to spare, I fought hard to forget what had happened and to convince myself that all was well. However, in reality, all was not well inside of me and I felt devastated and incredibly alone during that time. Sure, life happens, but when trauma is dealt with as it occurs, things are different than when it goes untreated for years, even decades, as was the case with me.

Traumatic experiences need to be dealt with as they occur or they will emerge somehow, either affecting mental health or physical health or spiritual health or all three. Had someone in my youth, or after the gang rape, helped me to deal early on with the trauma, or had I gotten some good therapy early on in my young life, perhaps the PTSD, depression, and neuro-immune infirmity would not be the intrusive companions they have been throughout my adult life.

During this time, while I was attempting to process [deny and avoid] my traumatic childhood, I strayed far from the Lord as often is the case with college students, and continued to drink in excess to ease my deep, long time emotional pain. I did not pray much, if at all, nor did I go to church. Clearly, it was a compartmentalized time in my life, as I was reeling in emotional pain, resisted counseling help, and had wandered far off the beaten path the Lord had prepared for me.

In essence, I wondered where God was in all of this, not realizing it was I who had walked away from Him.

Out of necessity I had, in my youth, previously always tried to stay close to Jesus after my mother told me about Him as a young child. Though I could not see Him, I felt that I just had to trust in His presence in my life. Though my relationship with my mother was difficult at best, her early Catholic teachings about Jesus, before she got sick went a long way to foster my knowledge and love of Him. In fact, by the grace of God, she fully armed me with faith in Jesus by the age of six before she went into the mental institution. She did so by telling me about God, Jesus, the Holy Spirit, and the Blessed Mother, all in one fell swoop.

For a time, I had walked away from all of them and I was tragically on my own. *But now it was my time to return to Jesus by choice.* But I had gotten so far off the beaten path, the pressing question was, 'How do I return?" Through too much trauma, I had traversed so far off the beaten path. Right after the gang rape, I could no longer contain my sadness from the early trauma. The recent trauma filled my cup to overflowing with uncontainable grief, shame and self-blame. It was at this point in my life that I wept bitterly and often as I grieved the many losses I had experienced in my early life. And I continued to drink with more fervor than ever before, in an effort to try to dull the emotional pain as it had become my constant companion, an unbearable feeling I was fully unprepared to deal with.

I did not seek counseling or tell anyone what happened to me except I called my sister, who I was not really close to at that time. She had been like a mother to me while growing up. As I recall, her reaction was rather distant and detached, and it seemed I was unable to help her understand the severity of what had happened. I remember thinking, if my own sister doesn't get this, how will I ever be able to tell the police and have them care? Because of her tepid reaction, I did not go to the police, nor did I go to the local ER for post-rape treatment or counseling.

Instead, I cried incessantly, and pulled away from everyone, isolated myself for what felt like an endless period of time, until no more tears would come, then I cried some more.

All I knew was that after the gang rape occurred, I was broken. **REALLY BROKEN**, and acutely alone, and it stirred up all sorts of buried memories from my traumatic childhood with Howie and my mother, Gina. I couldn't stop thinking that no one in the residence where I lived with 5 other girls came to my rescue; no one heard anything or came to help. Though I asked, none of my roommates came forward with any information or support. Reminiscent of the incident with Kay and the taxi driver in my early youth, had my roommates turned a deaf ear and walked away in my greatest hour of need? Though we lived in a big house, there had to be someone who heard or saw something. However, no one ever admitted to seeing anything or came forward to help in the aftermath as I struggled to make sense of it all. I came to believe that healing from trauma is a process, and it's how you do it that makes the difference.

Though what happened haunted me for many years, after about 2 weeks I forced myself to begin the process of putting aside the trauma just enough to get on with my pre-nursing studies, but continued to stuff my feelings as I always had in the past. At times, for decades after, I cried at the drop of a hat for apparently no reason. Though normally outgoing, having a kind word and smile for everyone, weeping in isolation seemed to be my preferred method of coping.

After some weeks, I finally realized that I had to be sharp and resilient and regain my composure; I had to be on my game if I was ever going to realize my childhood dream to become a registered nurse and prove my mother wrong. I had a tough, full 17 credit course load that semester that included anatomy and physiology and microbiology with labs for both. Putting one foot in front of the other, as I always had in the face of trauma in the past, I finally returned to classes and resumed my studies as if nothing ever happened. In a word, I was able to compartmentalize the trauma, hoping against hope it would go away on its own.

Again, with nowhere to turn for solace and comfort, I buried the experience far away from my conscious mind and tried to put it all aside and press on with 'business as usual.' Yet deep inside, my emotions fomented, and all was not well, as the effects of the trauma lingered and went untreated. After that fateful night, though I was unable to put it all together, my sleep was disturbed, I began to drink much more heavily, and developed an untreated eating disorder alternating starvation with binge eating and drinking, and cried often, clearly all emotional signs of trauma. My body and mind were trying to tell me I was in crisis, that I was hurting, and in need of emotional help. But the thought of the stigma associated with getting emotional help that my mother had instilled in me was overwhelming and loomed large.

Being new to town, I had acquaintances but did not have close friends. I'm not sure how, but by the grace of God, I began reading my Bible again and seeking God in earnest. I suppose that really was my silver lining. From that point forward, I tried to drink less, though unsuccessfully, and focused more on my pre-nursing studies. The ongoing prayer I recited over and over in my anguished grief, was a simple one, but very similar to my mother's repeated prayer of lament: *"Jesus help me!"*

With low self-esteem, nowhere to turn, and thinking perhaps I had somehow caused it, I felt so ashamed, and riddled with guilt. I never did tell the police or my friends what happened to me. I just felt so humiliated that I was fully unable to report what happened to me that fateful night when I was date raped.

Though I intermittently tried to pursue counseling, I never was able to find a good therapist match for myself while in college. The problem was three (3) fold. I never felt that the counselors I saw were capable of helping me due to my deep trust issues from my youth.

Secondly, campus counseling seemed to be limited to just a few weeks of counseling and I needed intensive therapy. Thirdly, my memory was blocked due to PTSD. I barely got to tell them about what was on my mind before it was time for discharge. It was 'counseling light,' but far removed from what I really needed.

It was not until much, much later, in 2007 when I was 49 years old, that I FINALLY found a capable therapist and psychiatrist team and started working through all that had happened, and effectively began the healing process. And what a blessing it was!

A New Beginning

Finally, one day, in late winter, just weeks after the gang rape, and about 1 year after my first recorded nocturnal grand mal seizure I had while I was with David, I had another nocturnal grand mal seizure. Shortly after, I made an appointment with a neurologist, Dr. V. J. Blazina who performed an EEG (Electro Encephalogram) in his office. The visit turned out to be a most needed God-send, as my doctor delivered a serious admonishment:

"If you continue to drink with your seizure disorder and epilepsy medication, you may not make it to 30 years old."

I was stunned but knew that he was right, as I was on dilantin and phenobarbital, neither of which should ever be taken with alcohol at all. It was a tremendous wake-up call for me, truly a blessing from God, that my doctor cared enough to warn me about my health and lifestyle when no one else seemed to care.

I remember going home that day after my doctor's visit thinking I may be an alcoholic and wept bitterly as I quietly wondered aloud, *"How in the world did I get to this spot in* the drinking had to stop, but it had become such a central part of my life. I wasn't sure if I could stop drinking, so I knelt down and prayed and asked for God's help. I prayed fervently that day, hoping that Jesus would hear my pleas and restore and rejuvenate me by helping me stop drinking to my demise.

And He did!

"The EEG test shows that the type of seizure disorder you have most starts in early childhood, probably around the age of six," he continued. As he spoke, I could feel my chest tighten and a flood of pressing questions whirled in my head, and I was speechless! I was 19 years old and just learned I had had epilepsy for 13 years since age 6 without anyone in my family ever noticing!!!

How could I possibly have had childhood epilepsy, and my parents not know it all those years???

I would have loved to have let my parents off the hook for this one, but the truth was that there was so much mayhem in our home life with Mom's mental illness and Howie's World, that it was highly likely no one even noticed I had a mixed seizure disorder with grand mal and petit mal seizures! Could this explain my early difficulties with reading and learning??? Why of course! Perhaps that was why I was often accused of daydreaming in class as a child, even in college. The night terrors in my youth? You bet! Could it have started when Mom went to the Seton Institute and I was alone with Howie while my brother and sister lived with Aunt Eva and our cousins in comfort? My mind raced. I was angry at myself for drinking, and angry at my parents for not recognizing that I had a seizure disorder, or getting me help for my early trauma. But now I had a new challenge. I had to learn to take better care of myself to avoid high level stress, drinking alcohol, to prevent or quell any future seizures.

Putting one foot in front of the other, I was slowly, eventually, able to begin to heal by decreasing the time I spent at *The Reef* and off-campus parties and was able to tapering my drinking significantly per my doctor's orders. Though it was quite a process, I began feeling better, more focused, more productive, regained seizure control, and became able to more easily walk away from heavy drinking. Concurrently, I got more serious about my pre-nursing studies once again, by focusing squarely on my goal to study hard and to try to get into nursing school.

As an aside, as of this writing, by the grace of God, I have not had any seizures in over 25 years!

I credit the Lord with that, as early in my life it was an issue but now it is not. We do serve a mighty God, one that can heal anyone of anything and with the blink of an eye.

St. Joseph's Hospital School of Nursing

After applying to several nursing schools, I was finally accepted at St. Joseph Hospital School of Nursing in their three year diploma program in Baltimore, Maryland, This meant I had to leave Frostburg at the end of my sophomore year, after being there for just one year. Though I did not want to school-hop again. I had already attended Towson State College and Frostburg State College. I was ambivalent about going to St Joseph's Hospital School of Nursing, but knew it would be a fresh start after the gang rape in Frostburg. I had grown tired of waiting to be accepted at a four year nursing school, as they were very hard to get into at that point and my GPA was average. My grades were not great, as my life had gotten quite complicated, and my learning problems were significant and in full bloom, yet still undiagnosed or treated.

Specifically, it seems I had difficulties with dyslexia, concentration, and focusing, and reading comprehension.

I decided to attend St. Joseph's School of Nursing in Towson, Maryland in the fall of 1977.

Gathering together all of my courage, I left Frostburg College, moved to the Baltimore area and went on to start my nursing studies at St. Joseph, a three year diploma nursing school. However, there were complications. Though I had told them I had epilepsy before I was accepted during the interview process, my having epilepsy apparently became an issue for them just one week after I arrived for my second year. Both Mother Superior and the principal called me into their offices to tell me that it had been decided by the administration and the nursing school medical director, that I could not continue there as a nursing student due to my seizure disorder.

'We have decided, together with our medical director, that you can no longer continue here at St. Joseph Nursing School. We believe that epileptics should not be nurses." Though the school year was just beginning and it was my second year there, I was told I had to leave, effective immediately. I had been experiencing some petit mal seizures, and though they were minor and not disruptive as far as I was concerned. However, they felt it best I go on my way. After going home and crying for three days over my discharge from nursing school, I once again gathered all my courage and strength and decided to move forward and to press on to meet my lifelong goal of becoming a registered nurse.

I have a three day rule: I can feel sorry for myself for up to three days, then it is time to mobilize!

Pity party over! If I was going to be an RN, I thought, I had to pull it together and try again at another school. That day, I called the University of Maryland, School of Nursing and scheduled an interview appointment with admissions.

I was eventually accepted into the University of Maryland, School of Nursing, but had to wait a full year to get in. During that time, I worked full-time at St. Joseph's Hospital as a nursing assistant in maternity. Anxious to get started on my nursing career, the year seemed to drag on. However, I was able to gain wonderful experience from working with the new moms there in postpartum, and gained some excellent nursing skills I could use later in my nursing career. I learned that no experience is ever wasted. Everything we do, every experience we have, can prepare us for other times in our life.

Though I had to wait a year to get in, it was well worth the wait. In the spring of 1981, I graduated from the University of Maryland School of Nursing, Baltimore, with my BSN degree.

Despite my still undiagnosed, untreated learning disabilities,

I studied hard and went on to pass the Nursing Board Exam the first time around. By the time of graduation, I had been married to Phil for two years and went on to work as a new graduate at Johns Hopkins in Baltimore in Pediatric Neurology. I just loved working in a teaching environment with children and their families, gained much experience, made many friends at Johns Hopkins Hospital, and treasured the time I spent working there, especially working in Pediatrics with children with head traumas, brain tumors, and seizure disorders, and their families.

Silver Lining
The Serenity Prayer

God grant me the serenity to accept the things I cannot change;
courage to change the things I can;
and wisdom to know the difference.

Living one day at a time;
enjoying one moment at a time;
accepting hardships as the pathway to peace;
taking, as He did, this sinful world as it is,
not as I would have it; trusting that
He will make all things right if I surrender to His Will;
that I may be reasonably happy in this life and
supremely happy with Him forever in the next. Amen.

Reinhold Niebuhr (1892-1971)

All of us have times in our life when we find ourselves in uncharted waters. Having found myself in uncharted waters in my college years, I sought God with all my heart in earnest to stop the mayhem I was experiencing, and to walk away from alcohol and to refocus my energies. Like the prodigal son parable in the Bible, I learned that God really is kind and merciful, always ready to welcome each of us back into His loving arms. I believe there truly is great power in the name of Jesus. Without Him, I would be a different person today, and very, very lost. I knew God had welcomed me back because I went from barely being able to keep it together to experiencing great peace and resilience and being able to press on through the turmoil and tears. Left to my own humanness, I seriously doubt that would have been possible without God's help.

Without Jesus, I believe I would still be trying to numb the emotional pain from trauma that I experienced in my youth and in college. Clearly, as hard as it was to hear what the neurologist had to say about my drinking, today I see God's hand in it all. In fact, He used my doctor to save me from my own demise. The Bible tells us that Jesus is the Way, the Truth, and the Life, and I, for one believe!

For me, Jesus was the reason to curtail, and eventually stop, drinking. I came to want Him in my life more than I wanted to numb my pain from untreated childhood trauma, and the rape, with alcohol. I needed to be sober to accomplish my goal of becoming a nurse, and drinking was only complicating my life exponentially. Jesus made it possible to do so, and I was able to embrace my new life in Him. I shudder to think of what would have happened to me in my early years and adulthood, had God not intervened and compelled me to seek him in all things.

CHAPTER 6:
Settling Down

*"This is the day which the LORD has made;
Let us rejoice and be glad in it."*

Psalm 118:24

THE LOVE OF MY LIFE

In October, 1977 I met and dated a wonderful man by the name of Phil Gill. We married in 1979, and 2 years later, I graduated from Nursing School at the University of Maryland, Baltimore in 1981. From a large Catholic family, Phil was a loving, caring, kind faith-filled man, and a lot of Fun. We enjoyed many of the same things. He was the oldest of eight children, and was very close to his siblings, parents and extended family.

Looking back now, I think I liked everything about Phil when I first met him. For me, it was love at first sight. We met at Hooligans in the Baltimore metro area in October of 1977. I remember being introduced to him by a mutual friend, and we talked briefly. When I stepped away to get a drink at the bar and returned, another woman, my roommate, had discovered him. They dated briefly, but she was never available to take his calls on our apartment phone (this was long before cell phones). So one day, I suppose because I always answered the phone when he called as my roommate was rarely available, he expressed an interest in seeing me. I asked my roommate if she minded, and she said *"No,"* so he and I began to date. The rest is history.

Phil is a handsome and tall man. He is kind, poised, supportive and gentle. He seems to be veryquiet at first, but is confident. From the beginning of our relationship, he treated me in an incredibly loving way. However, the main quality that set him apart from anyone else I had ever dated was his faith and integrity. These two traits have never lapsed and in deed, have grown stronger throughout our marriage. Best of all, he is everything my father was not, for that I am eternally grateful.

Though people are often attracted to and marry spouses with similar backgrounds, I love Phil for being different than any other man I ever dated, anyone I had ever known. A man of high standards, he was, and is, miles beyond my own father in character, and has Jesus in his heart.

Having been together 38+ years as of this writing, I still feel he is the kindest, gentlest, most loving man I have ever known, and he has stood by me through harrowing times with great loyalty and fortitude.

To this day, I really enjoy being a part of Phil's big family and visiting with them. The beautiful interstate highway ride to western Maryland is a scenic one, a trip we make often. I love being married to Phil, as he is a very patient, and compassionate man, hardworking and generous. Just three weeks after getting married, we moved from our apartments into a condominium in the Baltimore metro area, our first home. At that point, I felt like I was moving towards being successful in meeting my life goals, and my life was right on track at last. It was an interesting time in our lives being newlyweds, as Phil worked in construction and I still had two years of nursing school to finish before graduating from the University of Maryland and becoming an RN.

There was not a lot of extra time for us to be together. My nursing studies were all encompassing and intense, but we had dinner together every night and would take off on the weekends when we were not working or studying, and ride Phil's Kawasaki motorcycle in the country on sunny days.

Realizing My Dream

After graduation from nursing school in spring of 1981, I went on to work at Johns Hopkins Hospital in Baltimore, Maryland as an RN in Pediatric Neurology right out of nursing school, and loved every minute of it! I had really wanted to be an adult psychiatric nurse, but was told I needed 2 years of medical surgical nursing experience first. Though I was offered a job in adult psychiatry on the unit where I interned, I decided not to take the job working in psychiatry so I could gain more bedside experience by working with children from birth to 18 years of age. I did not yet know the magnitude of living with untreated childhood trauma, however, instinctively, I knew I had some unresolved issues to deal with first before working in psychiatry. Living with both depression and PTSD [yet undiagnosed], I was not fully aware of the depth of the untreated childhood trauma I had endured. At that time, my memories were scant. I gave my father a pass, so to speak, as the focus of my angst was squarely with my mother and her mental illness and cruelty. Mom continued her mental abuse of me throughout my youth and into adulthood right up until the end when she got Alzheimer's and died from a heart attack at age 92 in the assisted living owned by my brother and his wife.

The children I cared for in pediatric neurology had a variety of genetic syndromes, spina bifida, neuromuscular disorders, head traumas, seizures, and brain tumors. It was a really hard job, but very fulfilling and a great opportunity to groom my bedside nursing skills while working to help children and their families! Life was good while working as a nurse. Not only was I fulfilling my lifelong childhood dream to be a registered nurse, but I loved the feelings that came with helping children to heal. I really felt like I was part of a team and able to make a positive difference in the lives of the sick children and their families that I worked with. Often the children would come into the hospital afraid, and in pain, and I was able to help them become more comfortable.

My favorite patients were those children admitted with epilepsy, as I really understood what they were experiencing both personally and professionally. I knew what it was like to feel like you 'miss time' through petit mal seizures, and how difficult the post-ictal period after having a seizure can be when one is drowsy and somewhat confused about what happened after awakening from a convulsive seizure. I knew personally the embarrassment and fogginess that often accompanies having a seizure, and could empathize with both the seizure patients, and their families, as I had experienced them myself, and also witnessed on occasion my own mother's epileptic seizures, as well. I most enjoyed educating patients and their families about how to deal with the intense social stigma of epilepsy that was most prevalent at that time.

With over 100 different forms of seizures, I understood well how epilepsy could affect school Performance. Fluorescent lights can sometimes trip seizures in some people, myself included. In fact, all though college while in nursing school, I had to take tests in a darkened room, without fluorescent lights, as a necessary accommodation to prevent seizures. Most of all, I was able to help my young patients and their families 'normalize' epilepsy by encouraging them to live life to the fullest. It is always hard when a person—adult or child--feels that they are 'different' than others, especially when it cannot be helped.

My passion for my patients grew steadily and ran deep for the children and families I worked with, especially children with seizures, which naturally led me to volunteer for years with the Epilepsy Association of Maryland (EAM). Actually, I started 2 self-help groups, served on the EAM Board of Directors, and also was the Chairperson of the EAM Consumer Advisory Board advocating for people of all ages living with epilepsy. I also developed a *Seizure Observation Tool*, still used today by Johns Hopkins Hospital inpatient units.

Here I Am!

While working in pediatric neurology, I learned I was pregnant with my first child. My husband and I were so very excited to start a family. However, I had a high-risk pregnancy due to living with a seizure disorder, having to take medication to prevent seizures, and was experiencing high blood pressure. At that point, I had no other known pre-pregnancy health issues besides epilepsy and depression (the latter which was untreated), both of which I was able to deal well with. Little did I know the medical quagmire that lurked ahead. Hard to believe, but it was difficult to find an OB/GYN doctor willing to take my case and deliver my baby because I was high-risk. Looking back, perhaps it was a matter of eugenics, or the fact that they were worried about liability. They were also concerned about my having had a miscarriage during this pregnancy of a twin. The doctors we saw told us that I was high risk for having both epileptic seizures during delivery, and delivering a baby with serious birth defects such as spina bifida and cleft palate, in particular, due to the medications I had to take for the epilepsy. Various doctors I saw tried to have me abort both of my pregnancies. However, Phil &

I stood firm and would not even entertain the idea. We considered it unthinkable and kept looking for a good, capable doctor who was up to the job. After searching for several months to find an OB health care provider who was willing to take my case, we finally found Dr. Hamod, a wonderful Middle Eastern doctor.

He was a confident physician with a wonderful bedside manner and a supportive, professional staff who were willing to work with me. Even though I had a high-risk pregnancy, he did not seem to mind as that was his specialty. From the time we met him, we knew we were in the best of hands. His gentle demeanor and strong presence instilled confidence in us and we knew he was the one to deliver our baby. Concerned about my being on Dilantin, he deferred to my then neurologist to change me to a safer anticonvulsant drug. Based on current medical practices, I was placed on a medication called, tegretol. However, it was not without risk. The two serious side effects included having a baby with either spina bifida or cleft lip and/or cleft palate.

For us, having a baby was so important, but required a high level of trust and faith. Trust in the doctors, and faith in God that He would come through for us with a healthy baby. We prayed like crazy for a miraculous outcome-a baby without birth defects. But the hard truth was we had to wait 9 months in suspense to see what God had in store for us. Emotionally, I had to fight lingering depression and especially the 'what-ifs' that came with uncertainty every day. Time went by so very slowly for me on 7 months of bedrest, but Phil was extremely supportive.

Without many diversions, and the benefit of exercise and activity to produce endorphins, I found myself battling my lifelong depression and anxiety in new ways. It was then that I began to pray with renewed fervor. It was during the bedrest period that I began to learn in new ways what it meant to trust God with what was most important to me. All I knew was that I desperately wanted our baby to be born healthy, and I was willing to endure much boredom and emotional turbulence to meet that goal.

Before finding Dr. Hamod, the OB/GYN who delivered our daughter, I had one other doctor take my case, but only for just about a month before we had to let him go. One evening while under the other doctor's care, I hemorrhaged, and had what can only be described as a miracle. When I called the doctor, he did not have us come in, but rather told me on the phone that we likely lost our baby, reassured me we could try again, and had me come in the next morning for a sonogram. Well, the sonogram showed our beautiful 2 ½ month gestation daughter waving as if to say, *"Here I am!"* We were all shocked and Phil and I were thrilled to see our baby alive and well. Apparently, the doctor believed we had lost a twin in the hemorrhage, as the blood loss was not conducive to preserving fetal life. However, we had to fire the doctor when he pressed hard for me to abort the baby I was still carrying, citing my high-risk pregnancy and the chances for birth defects from the epilepsy medication I was taking. He also believed that if one twin had a problem or birth defect, then it was likely the other did as well. All we knew was that God had preserved our precious baby girl! At that point, after firing him, I had no OB/GYN handling my pregnancy for a while as we continued to search for a doctor who was comfortable taking my case.

Shortly after the miscarriage, while still pregnant, I continued to work, but the unit where I worked had an outbreak of meningitis. No patients could be admitted or discharged because of the outbreak. I went to my head nurse to tell her I could not work with patients who had meningitis because I was pregnant, and was told I had to work with whomever they assigned me, end of discussion. I was floored, to say the least, and concerned for my baby. Though I worked at a large teaching hospital in Baltimore, my having a high risk pregnancy did not seem to matter to my employer. This was the same head nurse I had earlier asked if she would order gloves for every room on our unit, as gloves were hard to find in those days, but necessary for infection prevention, protection, for both the medical staff and the patients.

"There is no money in the budget for gloves in every room." Was her reply. It is noteworthy that universal precautions did not come into being until several years later, in 1985, so most basic nursing care was done without gloves back then. To that end, not having adequate glove protection was yet another risk factor for my pregnancy during that time in my work environment.

By the grace of God, about a week later, after talking with my head nurse, my blood pressure elevated significantly, preeclampsia was diagnosed, and I was immediately placed on what turned out to be seven months of bed rest until the end of my pregnancy. I remained on bedrest at home, but was hospitalized the week before I had Caesarean delivery due to preeclampsia. To this day, I believe that the 7 months of bedrest was nothing short of another gift from God. Though it was difficult to be bedridden, it saved my baby and me from exposure to serious infections, such as meningitis, cytomegalovirus (CMV), and other hospital pathogens which were common where I worked. I basically spent my time on the phone and wrote advocacy letters for a project I was working on as a volunteer with the Epilepsy Association of Maryland related to current epilepsy driving laws. I also embroidered a Currier and

Ives needle point, made an area rug, and became an 'expert' on playing the game of solitaire.

Nausea was a daily visitor for all 9 months, and I could only hold down peanut butter and jelly sandwiches and water. So that is what I ate for breakfast and lunch each day. Phil would prepare sandwiches and place them in a cooler on the night stand by our bed in our upstairs bedroom for easy access. Some days my neighbor friends would visit, but most of the day was spent alone upstairs in bed per doctor's orders. It was truly a difficult time, but all I could think of was being a mother and having a beautiful, healthy baby!

During these 7 months of bedrest, I also continued to volunteer many hours writing letters and making phone calls from bed for the Epilepsy Association of Central Maryland Consumer Advisory Board. It definitely served as a wonderful, meaningful diversion for me while I was 'out of commission.' Later, for my successful advocacy efforts working to decrease the seizure-free driving period from 1 year to 3 months, I was awarded the Governor's Volunteer of the Year Award, a beautiful, engraved, silver chafing bowl!

Though I was essentially 'air-lifted' out of my workplace to home by God, I came to feel blest as time went on. When my daughter was born, she was perfectly healthy, but the 2 babies born to the other pregnant RN's who stayed behind on the unit working with the meningitis patients did not fare as well. Later, when I returned to work, I was told that one of the babies had serious bone deformities and a congenital heart defect. The other nurses' baby was born with microcephaly, a condition where a baby does not have a fully developed brain. By the grace of God, our baby daughter was born healthy!

And the Lord actually gave us another miracle…On our daughter's lower spine, right in the place where a spina bifida sack would have been had she had a birth defect from the medication I was taking, the Lord had placed a perfectly shaped heart-shaped birthmark. It was as if God himself had left his calling card as a reminder for preserving my pregnancy. Phil and I understood well the signature of God, and KNEW we were blest beyond measure for not aborting our baby! God had given us a miracle in our daughter, and we recognized it and celebrated it for what it was: A great blessing!

Almost immediately after the birth of our daughter in 1983, I became very sick just days after delivery due to generalized muscle weakness. It first affected my legs and ocular muscles. I tried to return to work just 3 weeks after having a C-section, but soon realized I was unable to keep up the pace and had to down-size my job by working in homecare which was not as physically demanding about 6 months later. But a medical diagnosis was elusive and I only stayed about a year and a half as I had untreated post-partum and lifelong depression with the moderate-severe muscle weakness. At first, I just blamed the muscle weakness on fatigue from having been bedridden for the seven months. However, with the passage of time, it did not take long to discover the medical condition was a life-changing one that would stop my career in its tracks for decades to come, and I had to down-size my job once again. This time, after working in home care, I returned to the large teaching hospital in Baltimore and worked as a charge nurse on the Maternal Child Care unit, including the newborn nursery. It seemed like a good match because I was not always on my feet, but I was only able to stay for about a year as my condition continued to deteriorate significantly.

I just loved being a new mother. Our daughter was such a joy. She was a beautiful baby, with little if any hair, but we bonded right away. She was a large baby due to gestational diabetes, and was nine pounds, fourteen ounces when she was born. With intense fatigue and muscle weakness, blurred vision, mobility impairment, and ongoing depression. My ability to function was severely compromised. Even going out with my daughter in tow was difficult, as the fatigue and severe muscle weakness progressed, initially, in my legs.

Traditionally, many neurological conditions are considered either medical or psychiatric; and I felt like the doctors I saw conformed their practices to that paradigm. In my experience, most of the medical doctors I saw initially were cold and distant. Though it defied logic, I generally came away from doctor appointments feeling like I was to blame for my medical issues, depression and later diagnosed, PTSD. In reality, they were compelled at that time to go one way or the other, but as we know now through medical research, the mind affects the body and the body affects the mind. There is reciprocity between the body and brain through chemistry.

Hard to believe, in my desperate search for wellness, in the first five years of dealing with this condition, I consulted over 70 doctors from various specialties. Office visit after office visit, each doctor told me they could not help me. Some told me to seek counseling or a psychiatrist.

Yet the dismissive nuances were loud and clear. One doctor even told me there was *"No help"* for someone like me. I was crushed, but it certainly did not make me eager to seek out mental health services. In essence, I felt trapped in my own body that had betrayed me, and it became a reminder of the periods of 'incarceration' I experienced at the hands of my mother growing up. Spiraling downward, each doctor that told me *"I can't help you"* brought me closer to despair and self-loathing. Between living with disability, severe, life-long depression, and unknowingly, PTSD, I did not have the power of positive thinking within me. Even praying was hard to do. I believed on some level that was where my healing would come from, so I asked friends and family to pray for me, and they did.

Socially, beginning with my family, it was the hardest time ever when our children were young.

Phil and I did not have words to say to them to explain why Mommy was so sick. I would just get teary and tell them the doctors don't know what was making me sick, but they are working on it. As for friends and extended family, that was even harder. People would stop me on the ballfield and say, even though they knew I was very sick, had difficulty walking, breathing and talking, *"They never did find anything wrong with you did they?"* It hurt me to my soul.

I grieved not being able to do all the things my friends could do with their babies, and turned down many outings with other moms and babies because of my health. This sadness permeated my days and nights, but I was, for many reason, hesitant to get help for the depression especially because of the stigma associated with mental illness that my mother had imparted to me in my youth. Early on, I saw several therapists, but never stayed as I had deep trust issues that became massive obstacles to getting mental health help, growing with each new practitioner I saw. At that point, I aggressively pursued medical answers, rather than depression treatment, all to no avail. Putting one foot in front of the other was even hard, and I fell often until I was prescribed and started using long arm crutches in the late 80's by a specialist at University Hospital.

Yes, the beginning of my medical journey left many questions unanswered, and I felt in a sense, like a medical orphan. After all, I thought with a heaping measure of forced false pride, I was a registered nurse. Nurses are the caregivers; they are not the patients. In my mind, there was a river of difference between me and those who were patients, especially those who were treated for depression. As if I were too well educated, too good to be sick and above experiencing serious infirmity. Little did I know that I had much to learn about putting people in boxes, especially, and including, myself.

In retrospect, some of the medical doctors I saw did try to help me, but as soon as they mentioned clinical depression, my wall went up and I would shut down. It was as if I could not accept my own mind-body disconnection. Looking back, it was in part the way they approached my case that was so alarming to me. Yet, it was as if I could only recognize a medical, physical answer for being so sick, but the answer was both medical and involving mental health issues from untreated childhood trauma. In truth, from head to toe I was a train wreck. Perhaps if I had recognized my own mind-body-spirit disconnection, I would have been willing to receive good psychiatric help earlier, and averted becoming as disabled as I was. But that is clearly water under the bridge now.

The fact was, though I had not yet been diagnosed, I had severe, untreated depression, complicated by post-partum depression, and PTSD, which was diagnosed much later, from my traumatic youth. I was sorely in need of relief, both physically and emotionally. Early motherhood was, indeed a very sad, lonely, teary time for me, and most challenging for my husband, Phil. I so wanted to be well, but the doctors were baffled and I was frozen in terms of receiving good psychiatric help. How different my life, my baby's and husband's lives would have been had I been willing to receive good psychotherapy and be prescribed the appropriate anti-depressant medication. Phil begged me to get help, but I would have none of it as the mental illness stigma my mother had told me about echoed in my own mind presenting a major barrier to getting well and my overall wellbeing. By that time, the muscle weakness had progressed and I could no longer work, or walk without assistance, and was prescribed long arm crutches as I had been falling. Due to severe, progressive generalized muscle weakness, I also had blurred vision, vertigo, depression, Cushing's Syndrome involving my pituitary gland, and problems with coordination and balance. Even my hand writing became illegible due to muscle weakness in my hands. I was very, very sick and simply did not know why... no one else did either. The severe fatigue and muscle weakness in particular, made it very difficult to function, but I struggled and pressed on to keep up with daily activities as a wife, a new young mother and registered nurse.

The Unpaved Road

One day, in spring of 1985, my husband and I decided to start looking for a single family home I came across an ad for a home in the Baltimore metro area, meeting our criteria, I arranged with a realtor, Bill, to see the house I had seen listed in the paper. As Bill & I stood on the doorstep in front of the house, a man opened the door. To my shock, it was someone whom I had met previously and repeatedly through my father, one of his close associates named Bob. "Bob?!?" I exclaimed with surprise, "Adele? Howie's daughter?" he exclaimed. In some odd way, like a déjà vu experience, he seemed so familiar to me. I even remembered his first and last name and his wife's name, but not the location of their home or the rural suburban street they lived on.

However, for the life of me, I had a sinking feeling, as I could not remember how I knew him and his wife "Dotty" by name. Likely because of my PTSD, many of the details of 'Howie's World' had somehow been blocked in my memory for years, decades, in fact. However, as the years passed, my father's local friends and their families seemed to frequently cross my path. At times, it almost seemed as if Howie was controlling my life from afar through other people. The answer to my severe, ongoing memory loss came much later when I began experiencing flashbacks and nightmares and was diagnosed around age 55 with PTSD (post-traumatic stress syndrome) from untreated childhood trauma. In a way, it was like living with long term memory amnesia.

Only in the past 10 years or so, through PTSD flashbacks and nightmares, have I come to the realization that Bob's place was, indeed, one of the very places where Howie often held his meetings with his associates in the 70's! Though my memories were blocked for many, many years, I often have had uncomfortable feelings about places I have visited and people I have met throughout the Baltimore metro area. Truth is, much has changed in that locality since the 70's when we used to come down this dusty, unpaved, gravel, country road in the country with few houses and no street signs to get my bearings. There were at that time, no real markers or signs to help me know where I was. With that said, Howie was usually very discrete, careful to avoid any mention of where we went—even as to what county we were in--and who he met with. I suppose it was all part of how he kept his world a secret for so long.

Due to blocked memories, I initially could not fully recollect being there before with Howie.

The road is now paved, reportedly was paved in 1976, though I had not been there since 1975 before it was paved, and there are signs, a street light, and many, many more houses there.

With the passing of time, since being recently diagnosed with and treated as an adult for childhood related PTSD, I have, in recent years, regained much of my memory with many puzzle pieces, places and events falling into place regarding Howie and his associates meetings.

Bob's place was indeed located where Howie frequently brought me week after week to recruitment meetings for his organization, and meetings in the 70's with his Mob associates.

The Baltimore metro area is where Howie built his 'organization.' With the passage of time, I realized that many of his closest 'business associates' and their families had migrated there from New Jersey, Baltimore, Upstate New York and even Takoma Park, Maryland. It is interesting that my siblings seem to have no conscious recollection of details from coming with Howie to meetings in Baltimore except for the fun places he took us--Loch Raven Reservoir, Rocks State Park, Gunpowder State Park, and Patapsco State Park. I, however, also have vivid memories, now restored, of Howie's associates and meeting places, based in the Baltimore metro area, and of course, Middle River, Maryland where he lived. This is largely because he was so discrete and they were not there as he revealed his double life to me over time.

Leaving Work on Disability

While other young moms would take long walks with their baby in the stroller, schedule fun playdates, go shopping and to the library, I tried, but was unable to keep up due to mobility issues and severe fatigue. How could this be, I thought? I was healthy before pregnancy, but clearly, everything seemed to have changed in a really big way. I was forced to literally shuffle away from my nursing career due to the extent of my disability, and inability to function because of severe, generalized muscle weakness.

For three long years from 1983 to 1986, I continued to try to keep my illness a secret from everyone, including my husband, Phil. Though my condition slowed me down, I put on my happy face when I was out and with my family and tried to avoid anything or anyone that would remind me of my infirmities or limitations. But the fatigue and unsteadiness on my feet told the story that I was unwilling to disclose. I diligently sought out medical care to no avail as I continued to go undiagnosed, while trying to avoid any mention of my lifelong, seemingly progressive, depression. Actually, being a mom and a bedside nurse, trying to hold on at work, and seeking medical help took up most of my time and all of my energy. There was little left for anything else.

During that time, I pushed myself to find medical help, but it was a monumental task. After seeing 70 doctors in about 5 years' time with limited if any results, I finally realized that this was a

"God job if there ever was one." I did not have the option of giving up, but decided to try and pray for a full healing. Looking back, I think if even one of the doctors I had seen had talked with me compassionately about the mind-body connection, how different things would have been. However, it is noteworthy that at that time, we knew precious little about the mind-body-spirit connection then— far less than we know today.

By August of 1986, about a year after moving into our second home in the Baltimore metro area, I had to leave work on disability. By that time, I was so weak that I was fully unable to function, unable to even water the plants in the front of our house with a garden hose sitting down in a lawn chair. Initially, I had to leave work on 3 months of short-term disability, and then it extended to permanent long term disability. Yet my condition continued to progress and baffle my medical doctors, despite best efforts. They were unable to diagnose my condition, even as it was progressing over time, but told me I had a 'progressive neuromuscular condition,' which sounded ominous to me and my husband.

The truth is, that some of the medical doctors just kept referring me on, and on, often to colleagues, because they did not know how to help me. Many of the medical doctors who suggested counseling were quite brash, disrespectful, abrasive and abrupt in doing so. I did not experience their compassion, but rather, aggravated frustration on their part as they had to admit they did not know how to help me medically; neither did some of them seem to want to. Other's told me it was just "in my head." I later learned that there are MANY women who have had similar experiences when they have what I call, 'The Trifecta,' clinical depression, autoimmune and neurological disorders. To be fair, complicated cases like mine are quite a ball of yarn to untangle for the average general practitioner, family practitioner, or internal medicine specialist.

It is complicated beyond textbook learning, and hinging on several specialties including neurology, pulmonology, and psychiatry.

Had someone sat down with me and compassionately told me about my own mind-body connection, I likely would have opted early on for anti-depression medication and therapy.

Clearly, coldly telling a patient their medical problems are 'in their head,' without offering them any real help or a referral is demeaning, and neither kind nor helpful. I guess that's why I shut down even more. More of an explanation is needed for many people in need of mental health treatment. In interviewing for my books, I have literally met hundreds of other patients with complex autoimmune and neurological conditions who say they were treated this same way on their quest for wellness.

Though I understand it was a different time in history, somehow my mother never grasped the fact that her life have been markedly improved by psychiatric treatment, and sadly, nor did I. The truth is, I followed in her footsteps to some degree. By her decision to go untreated and un-medicated, all of our lives were marginalized by her refusal to admit she lived with mental illness and get help. She had a similar fear of medical doctors, as they had what she called, 'the power of the pen.' I'm not sure that my mother ever realized it, but they were *emptying* state hospitals at that time, rather than trying to fill them, from the mid-60's on. And she had been a part of that movement when they discharged her home from the Seton Institute before she was ready to return to her community and family.

Anyway, Mom ingrained in us three kids that getting psychiatric care was the end. The end of your reputation, your life as you know it, the end of your freedom, and certainly the end of your marriage. And sadly, I took her lead in this difficult area of my life, by resisting treatment. I have grown to recognize that the mind-body connection is different for everyone.

People react to stress by experiencing sadness, anxiety, stomach aches, migraines, arthritis or other auto-immune conditions, sometimes flu-like symptoms or even neurological conditions.

However, everyone is susceptible to stress in some way, and we all have our own manifestations of stress that we need to recognize and deal with.

I remember many cruel, tumultuous phone and in-person conversations with my mother, especially after I left work on disability:

"Phil is going to leave you...what kind of a man would stay with a

woman who is sick all the time like you?" "Phil deserves better...He will leave you!"

My favorite was when she came to visit to 'help,'

"*There is nothing wrong with you. You just need to put on your lipstick!*" Mom persisted.

The afternoon after she left, I was admitted to ICU with garbled speech and severe respiratory muscle weakness. I was close to being placed on a ventilator, and they placed one just outside my door in plain sight. Actually, it served as a great motivator for me to pray even harder and get the rest I needed so I would not need it.

It is not surprising that I wrestled day and night with myself over getting treatment for the depression. In my mind, the depression wasn't life threatening, but my medical condition was due to respiratory involvement. If only someone had told me, matter-of-factly, that I had a chemical imbalance in both my brain and muscles; that acetylcholine was depleted in both areas, I would have understood. But my mother's admonitions about psychiatry swirled in my mind with the other old childhood tapes from my past, and I felt frozen, unable to take the 'big step' and get on medication and get some good therapy.

Somehow, I did not give up, even when the doctors referred me along or walked away from my case again and again without offering any substantive, real help, nor could I. Sure, I would occasionally give up for 3 days, but then I would get back in the fight for my physical health.

Silver Lining

I would love to say I was able to keep my health struggles and family life separate, but that is not the case. No matter how much I tried to dissect the two areas of my life, there was crossover.

Settling down with my husband and having children was the happiest time of my life. After having our daughter, though the doctors said I could have no more children due to Cushing's Syndrome, we went on to have a wonderful son. That pregnancy was, by the grace of God, uneventful, and bed rest was not necessary as I went into remission during that pregnancy. In fact, God blest me with nine months of remission during the second pregnancy. Our son was a big baby, born by caesarean section in 1989 at a bouncing 11lbs, 4 ounces! Today, our children are thirty four and twenty seven years old, and both are happily married to wonderful people. My little family is my greatest blessing!

CHAPTER 7:

Untreated Childhood Trauma: Fertile Ground for Depression, Autoimmune, and Neurological Illnesses

"Come to me all you who are weary and burdened, and I will give you rest."

Matthew 11:28

Beyond all the doctor visits, and the agony of not understanding my condition, beyond all the costly copays for medications and medical care that when added up, could have paid the mortgage on a beach house. Beyond the fact that they tell me this is a *progressive, degenerative* neuromuscular condition, despite all the odds, I believed early on, and still believe today, that Jesus is going to heal me fully one day. I am just on the 'Installment plan' for healing. One day I will no longer need the bipap respirator 14 hours per day, or to take medications and walk unassisted.

There will be no more garbled speech. It will be as described in Holy Scripture in the New American Bible:

> [31] *"They that hope in the LORD will renew their strength,*
> *they will soar on eagles' wings;*
> *They will run and not grow weary,*
> *walk and not grow faint."*
>
> Isaiah 40:31

Jesus has protected, comforted and healed me in so many ways over the years, so many different times in my life time. It is like I have been on God's 'Healing Installment Plan' for 35 years.

I'm just not sure when or how it will happen fully for me, as He has spontaneously healed me in the past of a Cushing Syndrome, a brainstem tumor, a uterine tumor, precancerous colon polyps, torn meniscuses in both my knees, PTSD and depression with medication, learning disabilities, a seizure disorder, healing of memories, and all the rest ... and the list goes on. Most of all, He has healed my broken heart, removing obstacles of unforgiveness that have in the past sprouted up in my life, making it easier to love my family and others as I should.

Sure, sometimes I lose my courage for living with disability and depression and PTSD, but then I remember that Jesus is with me, and I am not alone. He has a plan for my life—for I believe that EVERY soul is precious in the eyes of God--and when I remind myself of that, I am able to get back on my proverbial horse and ride, to press on, and move forward in my life.

Though this mind-body infirmity has been hard for me, it is no less difficult for my husband and children. Yet, somehow, we have been able to raise our children, maintain our home, and be a part of our faith community. Yes, it has been hard for my family, especially for Phil, but we have weathered the storms together well. I am blest to have good friends and family who helped with my children when they were young. I know it was hard for all of my family, but the Lord has used these experiences to make us all stronger for enduring it.

With Jesus at my side, I am able to wait upon the Lord to renew my strength. I am able to have compassion for those who have hurt me in the past, and begin each new day with a blessed blank slate. Each new day is filled with opportunities to grow in faith and forgiveness. There really is strength in weakness, and weakness in strength! Fortunately, recent advances in mind-body medicine today are making mental illness better understood, and the door swings both ways as the mind and body share chemistry.

In that way, the mind can affect the body promoting healing, and the body can affect the mind making it heal. The hard truth is that the body and the mind are, indeed connected in all of us.

This simple principle is far reaching, and has provided much motivation for the writing of this book. Like so many things, depression can happen to anyone, and no one is exempt; everyday people, along with doctors, nurses, lawyers, priests and ministers alike suffer with both depression and anxiety. The list is endless as depression is an equal opportunity illness—not discriminating against anyone! I think it is noteworthy that there are numerous famous people who have lived with mood disorders/depression including Abraham Lincoln, Vincent Van Gogh, Ludwig von Beethoven, Winston Churchill and renowned American born quantum physicist David Bohn, to name a few. The truth is that depression is no respecter of persons, and can affect anyone at any time.

Had my doctors and I understood what I am writing in this book right now, how different my life would have been! The mind-body connection is present in everyone, but every patient case is different and unique unto that individual. Emotional trauma is powerful enough to cause damage to both the immune system and the neurological systems. This is what happened to me at an early age. Infirmity in mind and body is also powerful enough to be passed down from generation to generation unless stopped in its tracks.

Untreated Childhood Trauma & the Depression Epidemic

When a person experiences depression or hopelessness, medical statistics demonstrate that the person is not alone. In fact, it is noteworthy that statistically, according to the National Institutes of Health publication, *The Numbers Count: Mental Disorders in America*, there are currently at least 20.9 million people in the U.S. per year suffering from some form of depression, also known as a 'mood disorder.' Astonishing as that statistic may be, it means that 9.5% of the US population over the age of 18 years old suffer from some form of depression. In light of these startling statistics, we can take it a step further and say that hopelessness and depression are rampant, even to epidemic proportions, in America today.

There are many causes of depression. For some, genetics may play a part. Depression may be induced or provoked by one's own mind-body chemistry, social environment, childhood or current circumstances. Depression may come with aging for some, or be experienced as a medical illness. In particular, patients with neurological and autoimmune conditions such as epilepsy, multiple sclerosis, lupus, arthritis, psoriasis, chronic fatigue syndrome, fibromyalgia, etc. are frequently also plagued with associated depression. However, in my experience, depression, anxiety, neurological and autoimmune disorders, and even addictions, often stem from *untreated* childhood trauma.

According to an online article 'Optimism and Health' by Rasmussen, Scheier and Greenhouse published in the *Annals of Behavioral Medicine,* June 2009, "Optimism is a significant predictor of positive physical health outcomes." Another online article by The Mayo Clinic also is in agreement, as it concludes that, *"Positive thinking helps with stress management and can even improve a person's health."* This same source also suggests that there are at least 7 health benefits that accompany positive thinking:

- Increased life span
- Decreased rates of depression

- Lower levels of distress
- Increased resistance to the common cold
- Better psychological and physiological well-being
- Decreased risk of death from cardiovascular disease
- Better coping skills during hardships and times of stress

In a study published in 2013 by the Harvard School of Public Health, the researchers stated that optimistic patients had higher levels of 'good' cholesterol, and lower levels of 'bad' cholesterol, also known as triglycerides. Similarly, a recent medical study of 6000 people presented by ABC News entitled, '*The Health & Retirement Study*,' showed that those who experience increased optimism have fewer strokes than their counterparts who are "worriers."

From yet another medical researcher, Dr. Dennis Charney, it is noted that optimistic veterans had lower rates of mental illness, most notably, depression/mood disorders and PTSD. For sure, guided imagery is another way that individuals are able to quickly impact their body chemistry as positive, hopeful thoughts can be psychologically and physiologically very healing in both the short term and long term, as well. Clearly, in light of these impressive statistics, it is easy to see that if a person is suffering from depression, that person is not alone in his/her pain. This fact has become a somewhat positive truth for me—as for so many years I viewed myself as alone in my brokenness! Today I realize I am not alone in my depression and/or anxiety.

Have you ever asked yourself why so many people you know are being treated for depression and anxiety or on depression medication? No, it is not your imagination. Actually, an ever increasingly large number of Americans, some diagnosed, some not, live with depression every single day. Everyone feels a little down once in a while, and there are various forms of depression. In my own life, I have established the three day rule. I allow myself just three days to feel down, and/or have a pity party. Once the three days has passed, then it's back to working. When depression stretches over time, lasting for three weeks or more, it is considered to be clinical depression, which indicates that there is a major chemical imbalance in the body and brain involving alterations in serotonin, dopamine, adrenaline, acetylcholine and endorphins.

Depression symptoms may include sadness, anxiety, hopelessness, lack of optimism, indifference to activities previously enjoyed, nausea, low libido, malaise, fatigue, sleeping problems, changes in appetite. It also may include aches and pains, gastric upset, migraines, and the list goes on and on. People with depression or mental health issues may also have unusual, long standing medical problems that may, or may allude diagnosis, leaving those people virtually undiagnosed for years or even decades. Individuals with depression may suffer with auto-immune conditions such as multiple sclerosis, lupus, myasthenia gravis, arthritis, psoriasis, or severe, multiple allergies, and a whole host of other conditions as a result of incorporated stress, and/or untreated, repressed trauma. These individuals may have an overactive immune system that attacks their neurological system resulting in neurological compromise as a result of untreated, repressed trauma. They may also have feelings of anxiety, depression/mood disorder, or experience Post-Traumatic Stress Disorder, also known as PTSD.

According to the online article, 'PTSD: A Growing Epidemic,' *NIH Medline Plus Magazine*, Winter 2009 issue: Volume 4, Number 1, pages 10-14, this growing epidemic is another serious mental health issue that often accompanies depression. PTSD, considered an anxiety disorder, is generally seen more often in women than men, and affects 7.7% of the American population.

Originally discovered as an outcome of direct military experience, it is also a diagnosis used for other types of trauma, including untreated childhood trauma. PTSD has the potential to run in families, and is the outcome of various types of emotional or physical trauma. It is often accompanied by depression and other mood disorders, anxiety, and even addictions as individual's use drugs or alcohol, food, etc…to try to help ease the emotional pain they experience post-trauma.

People may also experience a combination of problems, called dual diagnosis, a combination of an addiction and depression or other mental illnesses. Clinical depression generally requires treatment by a doctor who will most likely prescribe mood enhancing or regulating medications.

Taken daily as prescribed, these medications predictably take 3-6 weeks to begin working. Only the prescribing doctor can say how long an individual will need to take these medications. The length of time the medication is to be taken is a joint decision between the patient and the doctor and is based on the severity of the individual's symptoms, life events, and how effectively the treatment is working. It is vitally important for those faced with these symptoms not to self-medicate or stop taking the medication without consulting the doctor. Medication(s) may be prescribed by a primary care doctor, or a psychiatrist, who should be monitoring the patient for progress through regular follow-up.

When depression is complicated by untreated childhood trauma or is reflective of another mental health issue, like anxiety for example, and there is the need for more than one anti-depressant medication, it is imperative to consult a psychiatrist. There have been major advancements made in antidepressant as well as anti-anxiety medications and because of this medication management should be in the hands of a psychiatrist.

Today, many psychiatrists work closely with a psychotherapist, and have the capacity to prescribe a higher tier of psychiatric medications, when necessary. This is particularly important with people who live with bipolar disorder, and those with two or more other serious psychiatric medical conditions. Dual diagnosis, which involves an addiction to drugs or alcohol, and mental illness can also be very difficult to live with and complicated to treat, as can depression in combination with other medical diagnoses/conditions. These may require a psychiatrist with advanced training to prescribe higher tier medications such as Seroquel, Abilify, or even Cymbalta.

It is noteworthy that not all depression comes from grief, or complicated childhood trauma.

Sometimes depression can be part of one's genetic makeup, accompany auto-immune or neurological disease, or other times it may arise spontaneously with the hormonal changes of pregnancy, as in post-partum depression, or as a response to a specific stressful situation.

In my experience, looking back, post-partum depression for me occurred almost immediately after each of my babies were born, and was accompanied by muscle weakness in my arms and legs with my first Caesarean section. Post-partum depression is especially a concern, because it can affect the health and welfare of both the woman, and her newborn infant. In my case, the progressive muscle weakness lasted some 35 years and was accompanied by tears, sadness, and anxiety. I was forced to return to work as a registered nurse just 3 weeks after my C-section or lose my job. I had used up my leave when I was on 7 months bedrest while pregnant due to pre-eclampsia.

Moreover, what I have discovered, quite inadvertently, through interviewing people for my books, is that survivors of childhood trauma often live daily with neuro-immune infirmities and moderate to severe depression in their adult lives, but frequently only have a vague idea of why.

In my case, my childhood memories were blocked, to the extent that I was unable to clearly know with surety why I was so sad until decades later in my 50's. The hard truth is, that many people like me have deeply buried traumatic early childhood experiences and memories, that can eventually bubble up, and must be dealt with. If they are not dealt with in a timely way, these blocked memories can erupt, and can even become the cause of acute mental health issues or chronic physical illness(s), or both, later in life.

In retrospect, Jesus was with me by my side through it all, and he provided me with blessed consolation and sublime confidence in Him. I wouldn't say I have always been religious or filled with faith at that time as I did not go to church and did not walk the walk. But it was more a matter of survival for me to turn to Jesus when there was no one else to trust and depend on.

It was Jesus himself who provided me with the necessary combination of gifts of patience and persistence that gave me the ability to be tenacious and resilient during my early years, regardless of adversity or circumstances. Grounded in the understanding that every day is a new day; each morning a fresh start, God allowed me the privilege to be a child of hope, even when it clearly defied circumstances and logic.

There are special times in life set aside by God for specific purposes. I can attest to this, for in the hands of God, nothing is ever wasted. The Lord can, and will, use anyone and any circumstance for the common good. Every human life and season in life has intrinsic value from the cradle to the grave, even if to simply help other people take stock of their own abundant blessings!

Each new day is a blessed opportunity to experience the seasons of life, both joyous and challenging, as they present themselves. Let the seasons in your life evolve as they will according to the Divine Plan, and rejoice. There really is an appointed time for everything under Heaven. For in all things great and small, there is instruction, guidance, counsel, comfort protection and saving grace for those who but call upon the name of Jesus. It almost seems too good to be true, but this I know, when you humble yourself and lay it all out before The Lord, you will be profoundly blest!

"This is the day the Lord has made;
we will rejoice and be glad in it."

Psalm 118:24

Today, oddly enough, I am grateful for the childhood I had, even for the parents I had, and I know, despite their own personal challenges and 'demons,' they helped me grow in compassion and love, forming a solid faith foundation of my very own for future generations in my own family. Perhaps it was not by modeling after them that it occurred; but rather through the difficult school of life experiences. Like a tiny flower emerging from cracked concrete, so my unlikely compassion grew from the throes, the abyss, of untreated childhood trauma.

Despite it all, Jesus was ever present for me. I believed and still do believe with all my heart that He was with me and would guide me, protect me, and comfort me. In the early years, wedged between the wrath of Mom's mental illness and mental abuse, and Dad and his despotic 'associates,' Jesus preserved me even as I was placed in harm's way through the day in and day out of my everyday life with Mom after the divorce, and Dad's 'activities' with his 'associates.'

Yes, there was abuse: physical, sexual, mental, emotional, and, spiritual. Yes, there was poverty, rejection, abandonment and neglect. But it 'grew me' into a person of faith and compassion, at a very early age.

If this sounds familiar to you, I implore you to stay the course. Relief is on the way. Hopefully you will not wait until you are 50 to begin to seriously work on healing those old wounds like I did. I believe that the mind-body disconnection is a universal reality that everyone experiences at some point in their lives. It is often manifested through headaches, stomach aches, auto-immune and neurological disorders, and the like. However, embracing the Mind-Body-*Faith Phenomenon*© is a choice. It is a conscious decision to seek out faith as an avenue to wholeness and to realize maximal wellness in body, mind and spirit. Ask for Jesus' help today, and see what transpires. You have nothing to lose but the fear and anxiety that you live with everyday-- *faith and fear cannot co-exist*!

In my mind, the only thing harder than living with depression is when it is complicated by physical infirmity, or disability. Since first getting sick in 1983 after childbirth, I have become acutely aware of my own mind-body connection, as I have lived for the past 35 years with this progressive degenerative neuromuscular condition. This awareness did not come easily, but was hard won over time. In 2007, my psychiatrist, working closely with my neurologist of 25 years, told me for the first time that my medical condition is caused by damage to my immune and neuromuscular systems from untreated childhood trauma. In actuality, my immune system is stuck in overdrive, indiscriminately attacking my central nervous system neural receptors at the neuro-muscular junction. The result? The muscles are unable to get the chemical they need to work properly, and myasthenia-like syndrome has finally been diagnosed after 35 years. Before that, my neurologist was treating symptoms as they would arise with five days of intravenous Immuno-Gamma Globulin, or IVIG, a blood product. I received these IV treatments everyone tothree months for about nine years until my body got used to them and the treatment stopped working.

This lack of an accurate diagnosis spanning over 5 decades has been the source of great anguish and frustration for me, my husband and children. It has prevented me from even being able to join a support group, as diagnosis is required before joining. It has also prevented me from understanding the implications of my mind-body disconnection and joining others with the same condition.

After initially seeing approximately 70 medical specialists in my early desperate search for wellness in the first few years of infirmity, and enduring years of childhood-related PTSD flashbacks and nightmares from my youth, I finally realized that this illness was not my battle to fight alone. This was a 'God job' if there ever was one!

In a way, on a lighter note, this experience I had with doctors reminds me of Elaine on Seinfeld when she went to a string of doctors, all to no avail. They just kept passing her along and warning the next doctor she planned to see. Though I laugh hard at that scenario, her experience was not unlike my own, which might be why it struck me as being so funny. In truth, it is very hard to be sick, unable to find a correct diagnosis, a doctor who can effectively treat you, and subsequently, unable to find a cure.

Praise God I was finally able to find my current neurologist some 25+ years ago, after years of searching for a neurologist to take my case and help me, thus seemingly ending my medical quest on the medical merry-go-round to find a doctor to help me!

Dr. Scott and the Medical Merry-Go-Round

Once, during a neuromuscular exacerbation before finding my neurologist, my respiratory muscles became weaker than they had ever previously been, and my primary care doctor, Dr.

Scott, prescribed plasmapheresis. In this procedure, the patient's blood is removed and circulated through a machine, and then replaced after it has been filtered for antibodies. Breathing had become very difficult and labored, my doctor said something had to be done, that it was urgent.

Before receiving the treatments, however, he said I would need a central line placed in my chest in the operating room. A central line is a port that makes it easier to receive IV treatments. He gave me the name of a Baltimore area doctor, Dr. Smith, who he said was a good friend of his.

Though any surgeon could have performed the procedure, Dr. Scott emphatically told me that Dr. Smith was "the *only* doctor" he wanted to place the central line in my chest.

Although I was feeling very sick with garbled speech, labored breathing, swallowing difficulties, and mobility challenges, I trusted him, was encouraged that something could be done, and was eager to proceed. The arrangements were made, and we arrived at the hospital. Dr. Smith came into my OR room and introduced himself. I was prepped, anesthetized and made ready for the twenty minute operating room procedure. The next thing I knew, the doctor woke me up from anesthesia during the procedure telling me that he had nicked the jugular vessel in my neck on the right side, [the blood supply to the speech center in the brain] and I was hemorrhaging severely.

"Mrs. Gill, what do you want me to do?" Dr. Smith asked through his pale blue mask.

I have no idea why he asked me such an odd question at such a harrowing time. Shocked by his question and still groggy, I still had the presence of mind to know that the jugular is the blood supply to the speech center in the brain, something I had learned in nursing school. I also knew Icould die from hemorrhaging in that area of my body. I tried to say, *"Save my life,"* but my speech was fully unintelligible, even to me. In fact, I could not talk at all. I could only make guttural sounds. *"Do you want me to save your life?"* he asked sounding and appearing under extreme duress, sweating profusely around his mask, and from his surgical hat. I could feel that they were placing pressure on the base of my neck to stop the bleeding but I tried to nod anyway.

It was truly a matter of life and death, I felt, to communicate my desire to live!

When I woke up again, I realized I had been admitted to a hospital room. Three days later, I emerged from the hospital after this 20 minute procedure with a gaping wound at the base of my neck about 4 inches above where the central line had been placed. What the surgeon was doing up there in that area of my neck I will never know. The effect of the botched surgery was immediate. My speech was gone, and I was fully unable to talk for a year and a half after that fateful day. I could only make basic sounds—no words.

The plasmapheresis treatments followed shortly after placement of the central line. The treatments were only mildly successful. The nurses were unable to complete the full 5-day series of treatments that week as ordered. The central line was found to be infected and had to be removed. The IV nurses giving me plasmapheresis called the doctor on my behalf with the number I gave them, and sent me to the ER immediately. I wanted to sue the doctor, but I was unable to advocate for myself, as I had been rendered fully speechless by the surgical accident.

When I got to the hospital ER, no one had ever heard of Dr. Smith, and no one was willing to treat me, or remove my central line. The medical staff didn't recognize his name or even have a phone number for him, just the number I gave them, which made me wonder if Dr. Smith had physician privileges at that hospital at all, or indeed, any hospital They called him, and told me to wait for Dr. Smith to come in the ER. I waited over 6 hours for him to come. When he arrived, he seemed angry and yelled at me about my port being infected. But the nurses had been responsible for the care of my port that week, and given the surgeon's lack of surgical technique, no one could be surprised that the wound became infected. He briefly looked at the surgical sight, and quickly removed the 8 inch long central line with his bare, gloveless hands. He handed the infected, used central line to my husband, Phil, who was also not gloved, saying, *"Here. Throw this away in the trash can over there."* Phil complied. When I went back to Dr.

Scott, he yelled at me saying, *"Do you know what you put me through? You had us very worried!"* After a few minutes, he left the room and returned with his stethoscope to listen to my chest over the patient gown I was wearing.

*"You **know** I know your father, right?" "I've known you both for years..."*

"What!!!???!!!" I exclaimed in utter dismay with unintelligible speech.

*"Yes, I **know** your father."* At that point, after what I had just been through, I felt faint.

"Sure," he continued, *"And I also used to be the Medical Director at St. Joseph's Hospital School of Nursing."*

"I was dismissed from there for having epilepsy even though I had told them before I entered.

They told me that the medical director decided that epileptics should not be nurses!"

"I know. I was part of the team making the decision to let you go from that nursing school."

Lord have mercy, I thought—this doctor who ordered my central line was the same doctor who was the medical director at St. Joseph's Nursing School and he was involved in the decision to dismiss me from the nursing program. And he said he was one of my dad's close associates.

Looking closely at him again, I realized it was true on both counts. Words cannot describe how I felt that day. This doctor said he knew my dad well, but for some reason, at first, I could not at place him, or how old I had been when we had originally met, or where, though with time it became clearer.

Over the years, I have come to dread those four words I have heard so often with all my being:

"I knew/know your father." I stopped cold, took a long look at his face in hopes it would trip my long-term memory, but it did not initially click for me. However, eventually, I did remember that he was, indeed, the medical director at the nursing school I had attended. As far as I recall, I had only met Dr. Scott once for my school entrance physical exam circa 1977 some 23 years before meeting him again in his office. When I had met him at St. Joseph's he was muscular then, and had a full head of red hair in a sort of Afro-style, but now he was bald, portly, and much older.

The disparity in his appearance, combined with blocked memories from my PTSD, initially prevented me from recognizing him until much, much later as someone I had met in my youth.

Feeling sick to my stomach, flushed, afraid, vulnerable, and violated, I gathered my clothes, changed in the other exam room, and left his office that day as quickly as my feet could carry me, never to return again. I was incensed that THIS was the doctor who almost ruined my career by having me dismissed from nursing school for having epilepsy. Most of all I was haunted by his saying, *"**I know** your father."* Some years later, through therapy, I realized he was one of Dad's Utica associates. I had met him repeatedly, and his cousin, Manny in Herkimer, New York while mining for quartz there with Dad as a young girl.

Fast Forward

The above doctors are both still in private practice in the Baltimore metro area. I attempted to sue the surgeon for medical malpractice, but my speech prevented me from pursuing it as I was fully unable to advocate for myself. The slow-healing, gaping surgical wound at the base of my neck was healed completely on the Feast Day of St. Blaise, the patron saint of throat illnesses, the morning after receiving the anointing of the sick and a special blessing of my throat at my church.

Some months after the surgical incident occurred, I went for 3 months for speech therapy and was told I had "No rehab potential...go home and live a quiet life." Since that time, by the grace of God, my speech has been restored, except for intermittent garbled speech when fatigued and during neuromuscular exacerbations. As for the doctor's connection with my dad, PTSD memories of this man are in the process of being restored via flashbacks and nightmares. I know where we originally met in Herkimer,

Upstate New York when I was about 10 years old, and later again, in my teens, in the Baltimore metro area, as he often attended meetings with Howie and his closest associates.

I have also been able to verify that he was, indeed, the medical director of the first nursing school I attended in 1977-1978. But the haunting question persists: *Why do I keep coming in contact with Howie's associates and their families?*

Our Big Blessing

There is one thing that the doctors did agree on. Several physicians told my husband and me circa 1985: *"You will never be able to have more children as it is physically impossible due to Cushing's Syndrome affecting your pituitary gland."* However, we were blessed with a second pregnancy, and nine months later delivered our second child by scheduled C-section. It was a tremendous surprise to Phil and me because of the doctors certainty that we could not have more children. More than a few doctors talked with us about abortion, but we would have no part of it.

We had always wanted at least 2 children, and that hope had come to fruition when our daughter, was 6 ½ years old. On September 26th, 1989, I gave birth to a healthy, bouncing baby boy, who was eleven pound, four ounces, and twenty four inches long, and what a blessing he was! The pregnancy of our son was very different than my first pregnancy, as I had little if any nausea, and the muscle weakness went into remission while I was pregnant. Our son was a very easy, content baby with chubby cheeks and a smile that lit up the room.

The morning our son was born, during breakfast, the medical director for our insurance company came to my hospital room. He introduced himself, then went on to say I should not be having more children due to my medical conditions. Then he told me that they were scheduling me for a sterilization procedure. Since this was a huge, unexpected surprise to me, I told him to get out of my room. After throwing him out and threatening to call my nurse, he returned again the next morning like a déjà vu experience. Again, I tossed him out of the room swiftly and reported him both times to my nurse, thankfully, never to be seen again.

Though our son's early days with us as a family of four were pure joy, the muscle weakness soon reared its ugly head again. I began having trouble lifting him in and out of his crib and Sassy seat. So I was forced to use the stroller, even at home, during his early infancy. By the grace of God, I do not remember experiencing any initial postpartum depression, but the depressive effects of my own untreated childhood trauma persisted.

I had a wonderful husband and two beautiful children to take care of now, and simply had to press on as I always had in my youth. I had to keep moving forward. As the depression eventually pressed in and I continued to resist treatment, there were times when I sought counseling, but it was very much an ongoing struggle to try find anyone I felt I could trust with my life story and my health. I think I recognized that I had long standing mental health issues, but was frozen by the stigma in my mind. Sometimes I was more open than other times to talk therapy. At that time, like my Mom, I was very resistant to getting help due to the stigma of mental illness, and simply could not bring myself to take anti-depression medicine until sometime in the late 80's.

My job was being a good mother and wife and keeping my head above water and having a good attitude. I noticed early on that the better I could handle things and try not to be depressed, the better life was for my husband and children. And how did I come to that realization? They told me so! But there was a deeper reason, as well. On some level, I never wanted my kids to have to suffer living with mental illness as my siblings and I had with my mom. And with that thought, I finally decided to take the risk and try to trust a psychotherapist to heal.

Accepting My Own Mind-Body Disconnect

You can bury traumatic memories, as I did for decades, but they will likely eventually come out somehow, some way, through depression, anxiety, PTSD, medical conditions, sleep disturbances, headaches, seizures, auto- immune or neurological conditions, stomach aches, eating disorders, alcoholism, drug abuse, etc…and the list goes on and on.

"People who have experienced untreated trauma as children, are often much more prone to depression, auto-immune and neurological illnesses as they grow into adulthood."

Efim Weinman, M.D.

There is much written today about the mind body connection. However, most of us struggle to understand that there is some sort of a loose association between the mind and the body. In my experience as a retired RN, health and spirituality writer, a chaplain, and my own personal mind-body connection experience, I have long noticed that there is a strong correlation between immune health, neurological health, and mental/emotional health. In my mind, it is sometimes difficult to tell which comes first, as the mind-body connection is a strong and enduring bond that may foretell one's story of unspeakable untreated trauma childhood. All too often, people whom I have met who have auto-immune diseases later reveal they also experienced untreated childhood trauma. They just seem to go together.

According to Baltimore area psychiatrist, Efim Weinman, M.D., *"the immune and neurological systems are the specific physical places in the body where severe childhood trauma is often processed in the mind-body connection."* That may, in part, very well explain the high incidence of susceptibility to autoimmune diseases in adult children of trauma, including diseases/disorders such as multiple sclerosis (MS), amyo-lateral sclerosis (ALS), myasthenia gravis (MG), lupus, psoriasis, fibromyalgia, chronic fatigue, severe allergies, and the list goes on. These conditions are, for whatever reason, caused by inflammation in the body, also correlate with inflammation in the brain causing depression as documented through recent research studies.

In a published article, entitled, *'Severe Depression Linked with Inflammation in the Brain,'*
Medical News Today, Jan 29th, 2015, David McNamee, Centre for Addiction and Mental Health's (CAMH) Campbell Family Mental Health Research Institute, it is reported that "Clinical depression is associated with a 30% increase of inflammation in the brain." This new, ground-breaking medical research study reveals that inflammation in the body is associated with inflammation in the brain. This information is based on study findings published in the Journal of the American Medical Association, *JAMA Psychiatry*. "The PET scans showed significant inflammation in the brains of the people with depression, and the inflammation was most severe among the participants with the most severe depression. The brains of people who were experiencing clinical depression exhibited an inflammatory increase of 30%." That is, people with inflammation in their bodies often experience the same in their brains, causing clinical depression.

Yes, the body and mind are very connected, it is just part of our humanness. The mind-body connection is, indeed, a strong chemical connection. Some say *"healthy mind, healthy body,"* indicating that depression likely comes before disease in vulnerable individuals. But the reverse may also be true. In that way, it is possible to see that early, repressed, emotions and memories, anxiety, anger, feelings of rejection, and abandonment may run deep, even spilling over when not tended to the cellular level.

In accordance with medical research studies, when one experiences significant childhood or other trauma, and if it is not treated or dealt with, it may damage the immune and neurological systems and resurface many years later in the form of physical or mental health issues, such as severe depression, and anxiety, auto-immune disease, and/or neurological disease, or, as in my case, all three.

For 35 years the doctors have been telling me there are many people who are sick and go undiagnosed while living with serious illnesses, and I just happen to be one of them. In essence, some eight years ago, I was told that my autoimmune and neurological systems have been severely damaged by untreated childhood trauma, which is causing a serious neuromuscular condition myasthenia-like syndrome, that produces weak muscles, most recently weak respiratory muscles. Not surprisingly, in light of the untreated trauma, I have also lived with epilepsy (started at age 18; in remission for 25 years) and severe depression, again, long considered a mind-body illness. For the first twelve years of this illness, I was bedridden and wheelchair-bound, but by the grace of God, and with the help of prayer, that is no longer the case.

About 25 years ago, I was prescribed long arm crutches and a wheelchair for distances due to severe respiratory weakness and mobility impairment. Pulmonary functions testing revealed that my lungs are OK, but it is the muscles around them that are experiencing weakness, affecting breathing, swallowing, and speech upon fatigue and during exacerbations.

Presently, I am still on a bipap respirator approximately thirteen to fourteen hours per day for respiratory weakness, am mobility impaired, have garbled and slurred speech when fatigued and during exacerbations. My doctors tell me it seems we have run the gamut as far as other medical treatments to try. By any measure, these can be seemingly insurmountable challenges, yet that is just a small part of my story.

Finally, feeling unable to cope with my medical illness and the fallout from my untreated childhood trauma, I reached my limit and "hit the deck" so to speak. In 2007, when I was 49 years old, I fell into a major depression, hit bottom, and was hospitalized for major depression. It was a dark and lonely time in my life that required brief hospitalization, an experience I hope to never repeat. My doctors, family, friends and I all wondered if I would ever find my way back from the depths of torment to a life of normalcy. There were 2 reasons for the my major depression and subsequent hospitalization:

1. I did not think I could live one more day in poor health, as I was unable to walk unassisted, speak, swallow, or breathe easily. My vision was blurred, with double vision at times, and I could not imagine how I could press on. I was so sick, that I could not even read a child's book with large print to my own children!

2. Though I did not understand it at the time, I was flooded with nightmares and corroborative flashbacks from untreated childhood trauma. I didn't even have a language for what was transpiring emotionally, and just getting out of bed and through each day was an ordeal for me.

It took three hospitalizations in a month, and twelve medication combination changes, to help me pull out of the throes of major depression. Together, the mind-body disconnect in my life presented the perfect storm. Eventually, my medical team found the right combination of medications to get me back on track, and for that I am truly grateful. During this harrowing life experience, I learned a lot about myself and life, especially about my faith, from a wonderful woman psychiatrist at the hospital. My Middle Eastern doctor, Dr Hanita Sawhney, was likely one of the people God sent to help lift me out of the depression. Though she was not Christian, she recognized that I was a religious person, and encouraged me along by talking with me about my feelings, God, Jesus, and my faith beliefs, something often omitted from psychotherapy by mental health professionals.

> *"For our struggle is not with flesh and blood but with the principalities, with the powers, with the world rulers of this present darkness, with the evil spirits in the heavens."*
>
> Ephesians 6:12

Dr. Sawhney challenged me to let go of some things I held onto with clenched fists to allow me to reach for my faith with both hands open and to forgive those who had hurt me in my past. She challenged me in every way to reach for God's waiting hand, and helped me re-establish my connection with God as part of my treatment. Her 'way' was so life-giving. Before I knew it, my faith was being restored and I was able to pray simple prayers again, such as *"Heaven help me!"* and I soon regained the desire to live. In that way, she was a blessed life-saver.

Though psychiatry generally keeps faith matters separate when treating mental illness, reaffirming one's faith can be important to help people renew their belief in God during such harrowing times. When all seems lost, God will get us through our greatest challenges and obstacles in the most glorious ways if we or our loved ones simply call upon Him in our times of need. For even when all seems lost, Jesus will step in as only He can, and save us, removing us from harm's way. His unconditional love and mercy endures forever and restores hope to the hopeless!

If I could tell someone who is struggling just one thing, I would remind them, *"If God is for us, who can be against?"* For there is no principality in all the earth that is greater than He who is inside you. For he is not some far off, distant God, but rather, the One who is intimately involved in our lives. There is no problem too big to solve with Jesus at our side. The Lord is kind and merciful, just waiting for you to let Him into every circumstance!

Shortly before going into the hospital, and likely a contributing factor, was the fact that my mother had severely ramped up her negativity and criticism of me for my being sick and disabled. I remember one of my final conversations with my mother at my home the day I was hospitalized in an intensive care unit at a University Hospital for a few days:

"You! I always knew you would never do anything with your life. Phil is going to leave you because you are sick, just like your father left me. How could he possibly love you?"

I felt ready to snap, but not wanting to be too harsh, I said the first thing that came to my conscious mind. *"Phil Gill? He's crazy about me!"* I replied trying to defend myself, but that was all I could come up with. My mother, never to be out done and always needing to have the last word replied in her coldest, steely voice:

"Hmpf...How do YOU know!?!?"

Realizing my heart was pounding and I had started to cry from her cruelty, I fibbed, excusing myself from the toxic phone call, *"I have to go. Someone is at the door,"* After such calls it would take two to three weeks to feel my confident self again.

For 5 decades, I had held on to way too many secrets, and endured too much of Mom's wrath, and had stuffed way too much emotional trauma from Howie's world, for way too long. I had endured my mother's brash, toxic loathing and torment, and I had had enough. That, combined with being physically sick for decades, forced me into a complete emotional breakdown.

Essentially, my mind and body collided, stopping me in my tracks. PTSD flashbacks and nightmares from my traumatic childhood flooded me, and haunted me day and night, and deep sadness and grief ruled my life. I did not realize it at the time, but I was experiencing rapid succession flashbacks that revealed more clarity to what had occurred in my youth. Now I know it is called PTSD, or post-traumatic stress disorder. Crying seemingly non-stop, I felt like I was walking in a fog and all but stopped talking as my speech was so garbled and difficult to understand. I remember thinking, why bother—no one can understand my speech anyway!

Up until that time, I had fervently searched for medical answers and treatment for decades, but as far as working on my own depression, not so much, I was in long-standing denial. However, at that point, I had had enough and did not think I could live in this disabled body one more day!

Though I have long recovered from the despair, major depression and the PTSD is much improved through the help of prayer, therapy and medication, healing took time. Lots of time—years in fact! People who have experienced untreated childhood trauma, often come to a time in their adult life where they 'hit bottom.' It is not uncommon for people to experience a time in life when they cannot, for whatever reason, simply go about their way. That is exactly what happened to me. I was bogged-down daily by 'old tapes,' depression, anxiety, fear, emotional burdens, and physical illness, old emotional baggage, if you will. This baggage left me very sad, weary, burdened, unlovable and unloved, with little physical or emotional stamina.

Today, I personally know well the many, pervasive challenges posed by childhood trauma including feeling unloved and being unwanted, abandoned, rejected, living in poverty, and homeless, neglected and abused. I know it firsthand because I've lived it. As an adult survivor of untreated childhood trauma, I am particularly interested in its lasting, long term effects. However, not surprisingly like so many others, as a result of the untreated childhood trauma, I, too, live with what I refer to as 'The Trifecta' of untreated childhood trauma:

Depression/mood disorder with childhood-related PTSD Auto-immune disorder Neuromuscular disorder

Over time, I have been medically diagnosed and undiagnosed with Multiple Sclerosis (MS), Myasthenia Gravis (MG), myasthenic syndrome, periodic paralysis, chronic fatigue, all to be undiagnosed later. My neurologist maintains I have an auto-immune condition affecting my neuromuscular junction that he calls myasthenia-like syndrome that is yet undiagnosed after 35 years. However, early on, years ago, I was also told by two neuro-geneticists that this is a genetic form of myasthenia gravis, specific to my family. After 35 years of being undiagnosed, it seems highly likely that I will never know fully what this condition is or have a clear diagnosis.

It is noteworthy that up until now, my psychiatrist, Dr. Weinman, and my therapist, Karen, have been most helpful in identifying the causes of my own mind-body connection, tracking it back to auto-immune damage caused by untreated childhood trauma. They are helping me deal with the trauma, and heal as much as possible, in mind, body, and spirit. However, it seems possible that some of the physical damage cannot be reversed, but by the grace of God.

They have also explained to me just how the mind and body work together in a non-threatening way I can easily understand and accept. What happened to me should never have happened and I did not cause it. The fact is that emotional trauma from living with my dysfunctional family "up-bringing" has done very real, extensive physical damage, some permanent, on the cellular level.

In my case, my psychiatrist tells me I have a problem with not having enough acetylcholine and receptors at the neuro-synaptic junction in my muscles, which causes muscle weakness. My overactive immune system has damaged the neural receptors in my muscles. The same chemical, acetylcholine, is also diminished in my brain, which is the precursor to the neurotransmitter serotonin that is causing a chemical imbalance.

As the old Rodney Dangerfield joke goes, *"I was lowered [rather than raised] as a child."*

Hopefully, through this book, I can help others release repressed memories in order to protect, improve, and restore their physical and mental health. In my own journey, since 2007, I have worked diligently over ten years' time with Dr. Weinman and my therapist Karen to deal with the fall-out of what happened in my own youth. In fact, Dr. Weinman was the one who initially suggested the writing of this book, as a means of catharsis, and also to help others who suffer with untreated childhood trauma.

SILVER LINING

Without my Christian faith, I believe I would not have been able to forgive those who hurt me and subsequently, heal from the untreated childhood trauma I endured in my youth. In as much as medical research tells us that untreated trauma can cause physical illness, depression and PTSD, I feel so blest to be able to pray for those who hurt me most in my youth, and ask God for healing upon them, as well.

This forgiveness is something I know I am not capable of doing on my own, as I tried for many years, but the deep anger persisted. Some wounds are so deep that only Jesus can intercede and heal a broken heart and body. Research tells us, and I know from my own life, that anger and a lack of forgiveness can provoke and even cause infirmity. I tried for decades to heal myself of my anger and hurt, all to no avail.

Broken relationships, broken families, broken hearts, broken bodies, broken spirits--they all seem to go together. Today, though it has been an uphill battle, I look at each new day as an opportunity to heal some more~ physically, mentally, emotionally, and spiritually. Through this perspective, the power of prayer through the Holy Spirit, and this expectant attitude of healing, I have been able to find great peace and joy, and engage in sublime forgiveness.

I have been able to forgive my mother for leaving when I was six years old when she became mentally ill. I have been able to heal the wounds formed by her cruelty after she returned. I have been able to forgive Howie for leaving us in abject poverty to live with his other family across town, and for bringing me into his unsavory 'good fella' world. I have forgiven Howie and his associates for the abuse I endured while in his 'care.' I have forgiven David for his abuse, and the rapists from college. Most of all, I have even been able to put aside all anger and resentment and forgive God for allowing me to grow up in turmoil and tumult and poverty, and living an adulthood with mind-body illnesses. With new found confidence, I trust that God sent me to the right family according to His Divine Will for His purposes. I have also reconciled my own unforgiveness for those who have hurt me in my life, and in keeping with my faith, asked for forgiveness from those I have hurt along the way, as well.

Yes, for me, forgiveness has been a lifelong job--a career. It is just that important to my overall happiness and physical well-being and that of my family. Without forgiveness, there is no peace.

Without peace, there is no joy, but rather, bitterness. There is no greater joy than walking in peace and joy with Jesus, unencumbered by your own sins, and those of others. I'd love to say I accomplished this on my own, but I did not. God, my husband, priests, a psychiatrist, and therapist have all had a large hand in helping me see my brokenness, embrace it and move on, and for that, I am eternally grateful! I no longer live haunted by the past, but rather, live in the present while looking forward to the future.

CHAPTER 8:
The Mind-Body-Faith Phenomenon©

"They that wait upon the Lord shall renew their strength..."

Isaiah 40:31

INPATIENT HOSPITALIZATION:
ON THE BRINK OF DESPAIR

In 2007, after living with lifelong depression, numerous medical hospitalizations in the ICU and neuro-step down units, childhood memories flooded my consciousness day and night. Ready or not, I was forced from the inside out to face my childhood reality one puzzle piece, one mosaic shard of glass, at a time. I was unable to stand up against, or stem the tide, experienced from the PTSD flashbacks and nightmares. Depression had surfaced with a vengeance, and I was inundated daily with unrelenting tears. I was experiencing the same emotional torment that I had struggled with after I had been raped in college. When faced with trauma and pain, I have also learned that 'writing out my pain' is great therapy, in fact, therapy like no other. However, this time was different. I needed inpatient hospitalization.

I had intermittently experienced severe depression since my childhood, so this was not new. The depth of this depression hit me like an errant ocean wave-a tsunami of the soul. It was very much like the kind of wave that pulls you under and tumbles you around as you try to recover your bearings, only to resurface weak, short of breath, sputtering, and disoriented. I was walking in a thick fog for months, with little, if any clearing, and no sunshine. I found it difficult to think, impossible to move past the wall of sadness and anxiety that I felt. My life seemed to completely stop as the world pressed on without me. It was, in essence, a period in my life of absolute inertia.

During that time, I felt as though my life had all but ended. I realized that the time had finally come to seek professional help. There was no other option. Phil tried tirelessly for weeks to get me an appointment with a psychiatrist, but we had to wait several weeks for me to be seen before there was an appointment opening. Clearly, I had waited too long to get help. I was at a critical juncture and I did not think I could live in this weary, broken, disabled body one more day!

Every day I struggled with suicidal thoughts and I pushed myself just to get out of bed. The 'perfect storm' was upon me. I was incredibly depressed and having an exacerbation at the same time, laboring to breathe, with garbled speech due to respiratory weakness caused by the myasthenia-like syndrome. With severely unintelligible, garbled speech, I had all but stopped talking, except to my husband. Phil spoke for me when it was necessary. It had become just too hard to breathe and speak clearly; too emotionally difficult to have people not be able to understand my speech as it took incredible effort just to speak. Moreover, I had adopted my mother's perspective--her phobia regarding seeing a psychiatrist. She believed that they were to be avoided at all costs. My biggest fear was being forced to go to a psychiatric hospital like she had done. However, I had waited too long; I had no choice. I had procrastinated in seeking help and now both my body and my mind were in a state of crisis. The time had come when I had no choice but to get help as I was unable to function on any level.

After several ER visits for major depression and suicidal

thinking, Phil and I wondered why I was not admitted. Though it defied logic, it likely had to do with the complexity of my medical-condition. We realized that the medical system we interfaced with was extremely limited in taking care of mind-body illnesses at the same time. Those that we dealt with were not onlylimited in their scope, but equally sorely challenged by my medical condition. The doctors who Isaw debated rigorously as to whether my condition was medical or psychiatric. The debate was stellar, because medicine is primarily prepared for 'either/or,'but rarely treat concurrent medical and psychiatric emergencies. As the debates raged on, I felt like a medical diagnosis would be helpful to quell all the confusion and help me get the emergent care I needed during medical exacerbations. Actually, the diagnostic process spanning years was hard to endure for my hurting ego. Yet, it was as if I did not seem to 'fit' anywhere, and no one could help me.

The day I was finally admitted to an inpatient unit at a large teaching psychiatric hospital in Baltimore, the doctor had ascertained that I was suicidal, as I plainly told him I did not think I could live one more day in my broken body. But there was more to it, *"Well, I don't think she will hurt herself,"* the doctor said flatly to my husband while preparing me for discharge from the ER, yet again. Looking at my husband, he asked, *"Is there anything else I should know?"*

"Well, yes, doctor, there is just one more thing. My wife says she has been seeing and hearing from Blessed Mother Mary and Jesus." Standing up as if on high alert, the doctor then exclaimed, *"Well then, we do have a bed for her! I just need to make a phone call"* It was hard to believe that seeing comforting, faith-filled visions qualified me for admittance, while being suicidal did not. But it was true.

Though I preferred to keep that experience to myself, I did not try to hide the fact that I had had these religious experiences; these spiritual visions, if you will. In fact, they were what sustained me through it all. To this day I consider these visions as a respite, a blessed gift from God. Who would have thought, given the circumstances at the time that experiencing visions was the criteria if you will, for inpatient hospital admission???

It is noteworthy that he was going to send me home until he

realized I was having unusual religious visions *in addition to* being despondent/suicidal. It was as if being suicidal was not enough to admit me to the inpatient unit! Ironically, I was so compromised at the time, I was unable to focus enough to pray for myself. Yet through these visions, Jesus and Blessed Mother were very present to me in my great hour of need, and for that I am eternally grateful.

In as much as no experience is ever wasted with God, I learned a lot from being hospitalized for depression. I learned that our health system has a long way to go before it can effectively treat mind-body dysfunction concurrently. This dichotomy lends itself to a major disconnect in the treatment of those experiencing mind-body connection illnesses.

While I was inpatient, I was not even allowed to get my mid-afternoon respirator treatments as it was 'against protocol.' Medical treatment was not allowed. This compromised my ability to breathe optimally, but still was not permitted there. In one month's time, I was hospitalized and discharged three times with unrelenting major depression. The first time was at a large teaching facility in Baltimore, the second at a local hospital inpatient unit, and finally a day stint back at the day hospital at the large teaching hospital for two weeks. During my three stays, I met many wonderful but troubled people from all walks of life, and some very dedicated staff.

One patient who stood out in my mind was Rosa. She was an Hispanic woman, close to my age.

She was well-known on the psychiatric unit, as she had been a patient there, repeatedly. She was deeply troubled with depression and anxiety, and would rock and pace the hall all day long. One day, I walked past her in the hallway, and heard her say aloud while holding her head in her hands:

"I have nowhere to go. Who will take care of me!?!" When I heard this, I stopped to try to console her. *"I am homeless now because of my addiction. My children kicked me out and I have nowhere to go when I leave here."*

This is often what happens to people living with mental illness as they press the boundaries of acceptable behavior. Their loved ones become weary of dealing with the behaviors and eventually become estranged. Pondering her question briefly and saying a quick prayer, I replied, *"Oh, Rosa! I know who will take care of you... Jesus will take care of you."* She stopped short and lifted her head to look at me, so I repeated myself.

"Jesus will take care of you." "How do you know?" she asked with anguished tears in her eyes.

"Because I asked Him! He is with all of us and He takes care of us," I replied. Rosa's face brightened a bit, *"You mean you have been praying FOR ME?"* she asked in dismay with broken English. The truth is, I had been praying for her since we first met in the admission area some days before. *"Yes, I have. Here, I want you to have my Miraculous Medal."* Taking it off my neck, careful for the staff not to see me, I gave it to her placing it around her neck.

"It was a special gift from my daughter. I want you to have it. Now, whenever you feel anxious, just hold this medal in your hand and say, "Jesus help me!" Examining the beautiful, shiny silver medal, she began to weep. We hugged and she continued pacing quietly until they paged her to the front desk about a half hour later.

Within minutes she returned holding her new Miraculous Medal in her right hand saying excitedly, *"It's a miracle! My son just called. I am no longer homeless. My family will take me back to live with them!"* Though only about an hour had lapsed, her demeanor had significantly changed. She had stopped pacing, seemed less anxious, and more at peace. Her posture was much improved and the relaxed expression on her face revealed a new confidence. Two hours later she attended her final group therapy before discharge. During the session, with new found confidence, she departed from her usual quiet rocking back and forth to speak to the group, something she had never done before during her stay.

"I have something to say," she proclaimed boldly, for the first time ever in group. *"I am grateful to God for being here. Jesus has been good to me, and I want to thank all of you for helping me get better. I am going to be fine. I have a new life now and will be living with my children again.*

I am somebody now and have a place to stay." With tears in her eyes, she continued, *"With God's help, I am going to live my new life with my children. I will miss you all but I have to go now."*

As she walked out of the locked unit, she said *"goodbye"* personally to everyone, including me.

With renewed confidence, and new life in her step, I watched a smiling Rosa strutted past the usually locked unit door, while holding her medal in her right hand like a treasure.

"What happened to Rosa?" her psychotherapist asked as we waved her out the front door.

"What do you mean?" I asked feigning surprise.

"Something happened to Rosa. Does anyone know what happened to her before group?" she persisted. *"Lord knows,"* I replied with a smile, knowing that Rosa was in the palm of God's hand, and He was in control. In my soul, I knew she was going to be alright. Her depression and anxiety had dissipated into thin air, and had been replaced with a trusting, faith-filled heart.

Refreshed and ready to take on life anew, it appeared that Rosa had been healed by Jesus and was ready to begin her new life. As best as I could tell, Jesus alone had resuscitated her weary soul, and she appeared to be, indeed, for all intents and purposes, a new creation in Him.

Then there was Franco a suicidal patient who loved to play checkers. He liked winning, and I liked letting him win. There were other interesting people there on the unit, like Michael who lived with schizophrenia and bipolar disorder. He played the air guitar all day long singing Bruce Springsteen. I think he really thought he was Bruce Springsteen. Michael had a good voice, lots of energy, and was very entertaining, at least I thought so. One evening, while sitting with him in the day room, I got an idea. As he was doing his 'music thing,' I invited some of the sicker non-verbal patients to come and sit down with us and join us for the 'concert,' and to my delight, they did. With a little encouragement, and some logistical assistance from other patients, we moved all the chairs in the day room around Michael as if we were at a concert. Before we knew it, everyone on the unit was singing along to Bruce Springsteen, *"Born in the USA!"* This unscheduled activity was so inclusive and welcoming, we had even the sickest patients who had not spoken in weeks, some in months, animated, smiling, laughing and humming along. It appeared to be effective therapy at its best!

Needless to say, the staff was not happy, as they entered the day room and tried to 'keep order' in the psych unit that night. Demanding that the patients 'break it up' saying, *"We can't have this here."* Apparently, according to protocol, levity was not allowed on the psychiatric unit. But I believe the result spoke for itself. Perhaps, I suggested, they should have singalongs more often, as it brought many of the mental patients out of their shells. Yes, we breached protocol that night on the inpatient psych ward. Oddly enough, in my mind, and likely for all who were there, this unexpected spontaneous event became a blessing and a great, lasting memory during a difficult time for all who were there. I still smile and chuckle to myself about it to this day.

No Blame, No Shame

While in the psych unit, my husband and I talked on the phone daily, and he came up with a motto of sorts that was exceedingly helpful for my recovery. As I was lamenting about being inpatient and my feelings about it, Phil made a proclamation to me on the phone: *"No shame, no blame."* This saying actually became my motto as I struggled with, *"What will people think of me for being hospitalized with a mental illness?"*

His simple rhetoric provided clarity for me, made my inpatient time much easier, and made discharge home somewhat less painful. This motto challenged my own personal stigma I had long held about mental illness, the perspective I had gotten from my mother when I was young.

Through being hospitalized, I learned that mental illness, especially depression, can happen to absolutely anyone. No one is exempt. I came to appreciate the diversity of depression in that it can affect professionals and blue collar workers, every gender, color, race and creed. In that way, mental illness is no respecter of persons. Through my experiences, I have learned that everyone has a cross to bear; and that people, for the most part are resilient, and, even those in the depths of despair and despondency, can rebound. This experience showed me my own resiliency, my own ability to heal, and for that I am truly grateful to God!

One day, while on the inpatient unit, the staff announced it was time to call a friend and tell them where we were. I shuddered to think of doing this, and tried every way to avoid it. Finally, the time had come as they had given us a timeframe and it was coming to an end. This was something we were expected to do before discharge to show our readiness.

Gathering all my nerve, I called my friend Pam and told her where I was and what had brought me in there. Though she seemed initially surprised, she was most gracious and arranged to come and see me. She contacted our other girlfriends, and they all came together to visit me inpatient the next evening. It was great to see them, but REALLY hard all for all of us at the same time. *"How are you doing, Adele?"* someone in the group asked as we sat around the dayroom table. *"I'm OK. They are helping me find the right medication for my depression,"* I answered.

"What brought you in here?" my other friend asked, looking around the room at the other patients surrounding us in the day room.

I could not help but think how blest I was to have friends willing to come and visit and was overcome with emotion. I also thought how sad it was that some people had no visitors' day after day, and wore blue paper pajamas provided by the hospital because they had no one to bring them other clothes. It was as if the needs of those with loved ones were taken care of, the others not so much, which may have been in part why they were there.

"I've been sick for way too long, and didn't think I could live one more day in this body," I said tearfully, unsuccessfully trying to choke back and wipe away my flowing tears. By this time, I was far past stuffing my emotions as I had done my whole life.

I felt emotionally raw, and it was likely apparent to my girlfriends who came to visit that day.

Unlike my mother, who spent much of her waking hours and limited energy trying to keep her mental illness and psychiatric hospitalization a dreaded secret, I decided early on to be open and honest with myself and others about my hospitalization. It turned out to be a great blessing for me and others. That openness allowed me to eventually hold my head up and to not sink into shame and fear of having my 'big secret' about being hospitalized revealed to others.

Yes, having a mood disorder is a challenging part of my life, but depression does not define me.

Just like living through with untreated childhood trauma, the gang rape, and medical illness, depression is just another part of my life that has helped me become more sensitive and compassionate so that I can help others who are hurting, in mind, body and spirit.

Though tough times have brought me to the brink numerous times in my life, even to my knees, I believe that it is the cumulative effect of a difficult personal life experience that has allowed me to be able to effectively reach out to others in need. Had I not experienced the pain of my childhood, I might have been deaf to those who are hurting and who are in need of compassion.

For I know well the abyss of poverty, homelessness, and abuse; the ramifications of rejection, abandonment and ongoing untreated childhood trauma. Because of the sum of these life experiences, I am able to understand others, and let them know that I have been in their shoes. I am able to share about the practical application of prayer in daily life, and encourage others to pray for whatever they need with confidence.

Eventually after discharge from the hospital, I was able to take my 'no blame, no shame' motto to another level with a hint of humor. Whenever people asked about why I was in the hospital, I would simply say with a smile, *"I needed a tune-up!"* or *"I needed a head to toe make-over!"* Truer words were never spoken.

After two inpatient psychiatric stays spanning two weeks, I was discharged to the day hospital at a large teaching hospital in Baltimore, Maryland for another two weeks. When I arrived there for the first day, my third hospitalization in a month, I brought my CPAP respirator with me to help me breathe. At that point, fatigue was still causing significant shortness of breath, and subsequent 'fogginess' from lack of oxygen. I just assumed they would be prepared to offer me a room where I could get my daily afternoon treatment when I needed it. However, I was wrong.

Very wrong.

"What is that?" the intake nurse asked pointing toward my respirator.

"My breathing machine. I am on it about 12 hours at night and 2-3 hours every afternoon."

"You can't bring that here and you certainly can't use it here. We are not set up for medical care!" She sternly admonished as she went to another room to call my neurologist.

That was, for me, a stellar ah-hah moment. At last I realized that though we hear so much about the mind-body connection, there is still a strong dichotomy between the medical and psychiatric worlds. Sadly, the two are clearly separate, which only enhances the stigma of mental illness.

I was sent home that morning, and I was told my machine was considered 'contraband' at the day hospital. I returned the next day baffled by their lack of integration, but ready to roll up my sleeves to heal through therapy groups, classes, and one on one therapy. After talking with my neurologist, they told me I could bring my respirator but there was nowhere to use it. The staff bent the rules and made a place to store it at the nurse's station. Additionally, I was allowed to shorten my day hospital experience from 8:30am to 12:30pm, rather than staying until 3:00pm like everyone else, as fatigue set in daily and my respiratory muscles became increasingly weaker as the day pressed on.

Two weeks later, I was discharged from the psychiatric day hospital, I learned what a huge challenge reentry back to my life as I knew it could be. Altogether, it had taken about 12 medication changes to get the right combination to relieve the depression symptoms.

It was very hard to be alone at home after discharge. I ruminated over my plight and experienced great anxiety, but the Lord provided for my every need in the most amazing ways. My husband had already missed a lot of work to be with me before I was hospitalized, so that was not an option for him to stay home. However, I had an acquaintance-turned-close-friend named Linda who came to visit twice a day when I got home from the hospital.

She lovingly stepped up to help me get re-acclimated to being back home. Linda was one of my friends who had come to the hospital with my friend, Pam, and my 5 other girlfriends. She was clearly a gift from God.

Once home, almost every morning, Monday through Friday, Linda came to visit me at my home, ostensibly, 'for coffee.' This went on for many months. *"I'm coming right by your house tomorrow around 7:30am on my way to work. Can you have some coffee ready for me when I come over?"* Many days, she also stopped on her way home from work before my husband got home to check and see how I was doing, again, presumably for coffee. What a huge blessing to have Linda in my life, an answer to prayer, and clearly a gift from God for my healing. She unselfishly stood by me during a time when many people avoided me because they didn't know what to say after my psychiatric hospitalization. Linda's companionship also provided my husband with some well-deserved respite time. Looking back, I know the Lord sent her. She had so much to do with my recovery from depression, and for that I am eternally grateful! Linda even introduced my husband and me to her Bible study friends at the local Methodist Church, where we joined their small group, as the token Catholics, and we stayed for 8 years while we continued to attend the Catholic church on Sundays.

Fast Forward

Linda invited Phil & me to join her Bible study at her home. Initially, we joined because I really needed to get out and about more. However, we loved Bible study and came to love the people in the group. A few months after joining, I knew it was time to spread my wings and find a little volunteer activity and 'get out there' again. I had always been a worker and a leader, but feared that the stigma of mental illness would prevent me from effectively being able to help others as I had when I worked as an RN. I decided that I needed to put aside my own fear of rejection, and work towards becoming stigma-free, both for myself, and for others around me to be comfortable. Mental health issues can happen to absolutely anyone. Everyone has times when they need a little help. So, I decided to seek out volunteer opportunities I could do in the mornings when I was the strongest and not on the bipap respirator.

New Life: The Joy of the Lord is my Strength

Several months after my hospitalization, I interviewed and started volunteering at the front desk at the local senior center just to get out of the house. They were so accommodating to me, even with my walker and intermittent garbled speech. Though I did not disclose about my depression, I spent a year there, but continued to feel a tug in my soul to work with the homeless. All I could think of was how I had been able to help Franco and Rosa while an inpatient at the hospital. I have always enjoyed working with people of all ages and backgrounds. I felt deep inside that I was really meant to work in ministry with the homeless. Yet I had no idea where to start looking.

One day while going about my daily chores, I happened to walk past the mirror in my bedroom, and caught a glimpse of myself in the reflection of the mirror. I was startled by the extent of how much the myasthenia-like syndrome eye droop had affected my face and how I was aging.

Looking a bit closer, I became teary and realized that it was time for a good old fashioned self-pep talk. I remember telling myself: *"I am a child of God. I have much to offer this world, and my work here is not done yet. It's time to put aside self-pity, to stand up and make a difference in someone else's life now. There are so many people far worse off than me!"*

But what else could I do? At that time, my speech was often garbled and slurred, and my mobility was extremely limited, but I had to try and regain my sense of purpose. Putting one foot in front of the other, I took a deep breath and prayed aloud, *"The Lord is my Strength...Jesus I trust in you!"*

Soon, I found myself online getting the number to the local homeless day shelter, and making the call. With somewhat garbled speech, I set up an interview to meet the manager of the day shelter.

The day shelter was open to people in the community who lived in the woods, and those who stayed at the local emergency overnight shelter. I interviewed with the manager, Robert, and we hit it off right from the first meeting.

Before I knew it, I was volunteering weekly, fellowshipping and praying with the program participants. Occasionally, when I was up to it, I even served lunch to the crowd of 12-20 or so people. In the winter, there were about 40 people, mostly men, packed into the tiny New Hope Fellowship Church double-wide church trailer, all there to get a hot meal and stay warm inside, out of the elements. I can only describe this experience as life-giving. It was just a matter of weeks before I felt a part of the day shelter and was helping other people far worse off than me. I learned a lot there. I learned that reaching out to others in need is very important to one's mind-body health. We were not made to be lonely or alone; we were born to help each other. We were created to be connected in service to others. Though I was still going for IVIG treatments every two months, by the end of the first day there, my problems and concerns seemed to pale as they appeared to be miniscule compared to those of the people I was there to serve.

I learned first-hand that people do need each other, and that helping others is often mutually beneficial. I learned that my despair could be a great motivator to help me press on. Most of all I learned yet again that everyone has challenges that they must deal with. It is part of the human condition. I volunteered there at the day shelter for about a year and a half, then had to leave as my health could not sustain the schedule I was on when I had yet another exacerbation of my neuromuscular condition. Also, the neighborhood where the day shelter was seemed to be getting more dangerous by the day with much gang activity and increased, frequent homicides. It broke my heart to leave, but I could see it was time to stop going there due to health and safety concerns.

While volunteering there, I was happily distracted from my own issues through helping others, and did not have time, or the inclination, to feel sorry for myself. Most of all I learned that action trumps self-pity! The job was very hard but rewarding and many people I worked with, over time, by the grace of God, for the glory of God, came to accept Jesus as their Lord and Savior.

However, it was time to move on, so I looked for another ministry opportunity.

One day, my friend, Sue, visited and asked me if I could

substitute for her at the local soup kitchen while she went away for a few months with her husband to Florida. Soon after, I began volunteering at the local soup kitchen every Wednesday morning. Originally starting as a prayer team member, I would go table to table while the people were having lunch and gather prayer requests. People from every walk of life came to the soup kitchen asking for prayers for healing, financial stability, prayers for relationships, prayers for employment, and the requests grew…Each week, we had between seventy five and one hundred and twenty people who came from miles around for a hot lunch, a church service, and a free bag of food. Some came to the soup kitchen because they were elderly and in need of companionship and food, others were among the working poor in need of a hot meal for sustenance. Yet others lived in the woods in tents and without tents, or in their cars or were just out of jail. Others just came for fellowship and catch up with friends. The authenticity and diversity there is refreshing, and continues to lift my own spirits.

When Sue returned, she asked if I'd like to stay on with prayer team, and I was thrilled. To date, I have been there for seven years, and just love it. It has been such a life-giving experience, as I have been able to put aside my own life and health 'distractions,' and focus squarely on bringing each person who comes there, into the fullness of God's love. I consider it pure joy and a privilege to be able to be a part of the prayer team there, and look forward to it each week.

Wheelchair Time

In May of 2015, I realized that the medical IVIG therapy treatments I had been receiving for eight years had stopped working. It was, indeed, a scary time for my husband and me as walking, breathing and speaking had become more difficult due to increased respiratory muscle weakness in my trunk. The fear of being bedridden again loomed large, and that fear was large enough to consume me. So, I went to see my longtime pulmonologist.

Why are you here today?" he asked. With garbled speech and difficulty breathing, I tried to tell him why I was there, to no avail. My sister was with me and acted as my interpreter. *"How did you get in here today?"* he asked. *"I walked in from the car"* I said with shortness of breath and very garbled and slurred speech.

"That is not how you are leaving here today. It's wheelchair time. You are so short of breath that it is making it hard for you to even speak. You are too sick today to do pulmonary functions testing. Perhaps we can schedule for next week. For today, I want you to go to the hospital for a blood gas test." My sister completed answering his questions, and I left the office in a wheelchair per his insistence. Imagine being too sick for pulmonary functions testing. I had never heard of such a thing!

Wheelchair time? At first I felt indignant, then devastated, angry and fearful the more I thought about the ramifications of being in the wheelchair. I had been wheelchair-bound many years ago and knew well what it meant and how restrictive it was. I went home and had my husband get my wheel chair up from the basement, dusted it off, and used it from that point forward whenever I went out of my home for energy conservation. I did not use it inside my home as I wanted to keep up the muscle strength I had. Instead, I struggled to use just my walker in the house. I did soon learn that using the wheelchair when I was out allowed me the privilege to prevent falling, breathe easier, and maintain clear, un-garbled speech.

Giving up is not an option for me, though in recent years, medical issues seemed to be progressing in the wrong direction, as many physical functions have been affected includingwalking, doing steps, sitting for long periods without a backrest, using my hands due to contractures in both hands, lifting, speech [speaking becomes garbled after standing for several minutes], and difficulty swallowing when fatigued. Most recently, and most importantly, even breathing had become more difficult due to respiratory muscle/core weakness.

The next week, I went to my long-time neurologist, who told me there were no treatments left to try for this progressive neuromuscular condition. We had utilized all medical options over the past 25+ years that he had been seeing me in the office, and he concurred with the pulmonologist that it was wheelchair time. I was shell shocked at the idea that there was no more help for me, so I requested a referral to the University Neuromuscular Clinic. Cautiously hopeful, I had to wait until the end of the summer to get an appointment. I never really embraced the "wheelchair time" idea, and though it defies logic, instead, I started praying for a full miracle. I also continued to use the bipap respirator 13-15 hours per day, which helped my respiratory muscles rest while on it. The bipap machine provided mechanical ventilation to allow my respiratory muscles to rest. However, I did the best I could, putting aside my chagrin, while just trying to listen to my body and follow doctor's orders.

I was mortified, and could not believe what I was hearing. Though my longtime neurologist is a fine and capable doctor, I was referred to Dr. Pinckney at a Neuromuscular Clinic in Baltimore, Maryland for evaluation as I was told there was nothing more medically that could be done for me by my local doctors as my condition was progressing. Looking back, this seemed to be a milestone or watershed opportunity to get a consult there, a major step in truly discovering how to deal with my neuromuscular condition. I remember thinking it was, indeed, a new beginning!

Meanwhile, I continued to have many accelerated health challenges, a full-blown exacerbation, that included increased difficulty breathing, swallowing, speaking, blurred vision, and contractures in my hands that made them hard to use. As first prescribed by my pulmonologist, I began using a wheelchair for distance-walking as the muscles in my lungs and trunk were very weak. Clearly, the disease seemed to be progressing. It was a scary time for me and my family, wedged between needing a wheelchair, being short of breath much of the time, having to stay close to home with my Bipap respirator to breathe, and having garbled speech. I could not walk and talk or talk and breathe at the same time.

Despite how it appeared, there was no way I could envision this being the end of the road for me.

I refused to believe that this was the plan that God had for my life. So I stepped up my prayer efforts and asked friends and family to pray for me, and with me, while facing the fact that there was reportedly no other treatment to be had, which I also did not accept. I allowed myself a teary, well-deserved three-day-pity-party, and at the end of three days I was ready to pray harder than ever before for a full healing. I put on my happy face once again, tried to follow doctor's orders to the letter, and waited to go to the neuromuscular clinic at the end of the summer when I was finally able to get an appointment. It was a long, difficult summer in the wheelchair, but prayer helped me stay hopeful. I just kept telling myself, *"this, too shall pass,"* and prayed through each day with the understanding that *"With God all things are possible."*

Feeling rather anxious and sad at the declaration of 'wheelchair time,' I once again immersed myself in fervent prayer both personally, and also by asking family and friends for intercessory prayer. I began praying more often than previously for my own mind-body-spirit healing. I reminded myself that through fervent prayer in the past, the Lord has time and again led me away from fear and into a greater confidence in His saving, healing power. He has given me peace and joy during extreme circumstances. And this time was no exception. Though medically my condition has had many ups and downs, physically, emotionally, and spiritually, I no longer felt alone on my journey with Jesus at my side, and looked forward to what the Lord had in store for me next.

Another Chance

With garbled, unintelligible speech, I tried repeatedly, but unsuccessfully, to set up an appointment with Dr. Pinckney, at the neuromuscular clinic. Apparently it is a very busy place, and it took numerous attempts to get the appointment. Ultimately I had to have a friend complete the task due to my speech issues. The appointment was finally made and I looked forward to seeing Dr. Pinckney. When I went to the appointment at the end of August 2015, I saw Dr.

Pinckney, whom I had seen for the first time about 25 years ago. He is an acute care neurologist at a large teaching hospital in Baltimore.

Shortly after we exchanged greetings, he asked me to get up on the examining table and asked my husband to leave the room. *"Mrs. Gill, I need to ask you some questions..."* he said pulling up a chair. *"Did you have a traumatic childhood?"* He inquired. I was shocked, but felt prepared for almost anything. *"Yes, I did." "I have PTSD from my childhood,"* I replied hesitantly, unsure about the reason for his question. *"Why do you ask?"* He continued on, *"because sometimes PTSD can complicate these things [muscle conditions.]"* Sitting back in his chair, running his hand over the top of his head, he continued, *"What happened to you? I need to know so I can help you. Take your time, I've got time."*

Quite startled by his candor, I swallowed hard and struggled to answer his question as the answers to his question were rather difficult to explain and complicated. He was the first doctor to ever ask me directly in such a compassionate manner. *"Well, it wasn't just one event. It was ongoing. My mother suffered with acute mental illness and was psychotic most of the time. She went away to a mental institution for a year and a half when I was 6 years old. After she was discharged, she went untreated, and was psychotic most of the time. I believe she had progressed to paranoid schizophrenia, but am not sure as she was untreated after discharge. My father was in the Syndicate, the American Mafia, working closely with the Italian Mafia. Do you know Meyer Lansky, the founder of the Syndicate, also known as the American Mafia? He was my father's mentor. I was introduced to him as "Uncle Meyer" when I was about 5 years old while visiting Saratoga Springs, New York. My father worked closely with the Mafia, and used to take me with him on business. I saw and heard a lot, way too much."*

"Through these experiences, as a result of associated untreated childhood trauma, I have spent the last 9 years having frequent nightmares and flashbacks related to my childhood. I have been treated for major depression/mood disorder, and childhood-based PTSD, as well as, a myasthenia-like syndrome for the last 35 years."

"OH–MY–GOD" He said, emphasizing each word, while running his hand over the top of his head again. It was as if Dr. Pinckney had an "ah-ha moment."

"Mrs. Gill, you have two REALLY big problems. Depression with PTSD, and myasthenic syndrome. Normally we either treat neurologically

or *psychiatrically, but due to your depression and PTSD, we are going to treat both. I think I can help you get out of the wheelchair, but it will take time and baby steps, so you don't end up in ICU. It could take about a year."*

This was music to my ears, as I hadn't embraced the idea of being in the wheelchair. Based on his questions, it was highly likely he had spoken with my former neurologist. He went on to suggest I begin doing what I had been told NOT to do over the past 33 years--begin an exercise program for strengthening. With disarming candor and compassion, he gave me both hope, and direction, and I felt energized by the office visit. I was thrilled at both the thought of getting out of the wheelchair, and the fact that someone thought they could help me and get positive results. The appointment ended with him giving me his office cell number, something I had never experienced before with my medical doctors. I was doubtful I would ever use it, but it helped me know he was invested in helping me regain my health. Years ago several other medical doctors had tried to talk with me about my depression, all to no avail because I could not embrace, or accept, the concept. It was never explained before in such a kind and compassionate way by any other medical doctor besides my present psychiatrist and therapist. The last time I was told about the mind-body connection by a medical doctor at a different neuromuscular clinic some 25 years ago, I cried all the way home feeling that this condition was somehow my fault.

Today, I know better. The mind and the body are, indeed connected. Everyone has mind-body conditions at times. As my psychiatrist Dr. Efim Weinman had told me previously, I have a well-controlled chemical imbalance treated with medication. However, the same chemical missing in my muscles is also missing in my brain.

Indeed, I prayed fervently before this appointment, as did my husband and friends, for a good outcome from the visit to see Dr. Pinckney. I truly believe God was leading me to see Dr.

Pinckney, and now felt I understood why. He even agreed to call my previous neurologist, and my psychiatrist, so we are all on the same page. What a rarity these days; a true blessing, and answer to prayer!

After seeing Dr. Pinckney for the first visit, I went home and set up an Excel activity roster with stretching, leg exercises, using a core ball, and walking with incremental increases in activity, including doing stairs. By taking it slowly due to very weak respiratory muscles, I worked diligently on my program and started to feel stronger over time. The past summer had been a difficult one as I grappled with the logistics of having to be in the wheelchair, but this summer seemed different. Could it be this medical odyssey was coming to an end?

I planned to return in 4 months so he could assess my 'new normal' baseline. After starting the exercise treatments, I began getting stronger and had more stamina. Respiratory weakness with shortness of breath continued, but I was very encouraged by the progress I was making one day at a time. My breathing was more difficult during and after exercise and later in the day, but I watched it closely.

I first saw Dr. Pinkney in August 2015 as he helped me to slowly work my way out of the wheelchair to the walker by taking baby steps. About 2 months later, I started walking with a small group of friends, and was eventually able to walk up to 1 mile per day, 3-4 days a week with just a cane!

Fast Forward

I scheduled a second clinic appointment to see Dr. Pinckney 4 months later in December, 2015, to update him on my medical progress. He seemed very happy with my progress. However, it was at that second visit, after I got into my car and read the clinic visit overview papers that I got a big surprise–Dr. Pinckney had changed my diagnosis from myasthenic syndrome to "Chronic Fatigue Syndrome with dyspnea" (difficulty breathing) without even telling me. This came as such a big surprise to me that I called him to discuss it after I reading it on my office visit summary.

From my perspective, a diagnosis of chronic fatigue didn't even touch what I was experiencing and had endured over the past 35 years. I felt it was a nondescript diagnosis that could prevent me from getting the medical care I may need in in an emergency and during exacerbations when my respiratory muscles are weakened. However, he stood firmly behind his new diagnosis. I had wondered why his second exam seemed so much less thorough than the first visit. Could it be my new neurologist, Dr. Pinckney, was treating me for PTSD and depression alone–mental health issues–rather than the neuro-immune condition we previously had discussed? I knew I had to address it at my next visit.

"I was surprised by your giving me a new diagnosis without saying anything about it to me at my last visit. You may be more right than you know. I researched chronic fatigue syndrome and it is now commonly paired with something called myalgic encephalopathy (CFS-ME) which is caused by an infection of the brain, often infections such as meningitis or Epstein-Barr virus. As a nurse, I had high exposure to both when the unit I worked on was quarantined when I was pregnant just before getting sick in 1983. Three nurses on our unit were pregnant at the same time, but I am the only one who had a normal baby because I was home on leave on bedrest." Clearly, he did not see any connection at all.

"The new diagnosis stands," he replied matter-of-factly, without any further explanation.

Feeling like the winds had changed and he was not taking my condition seriously, I hung up the phone and pondered, *"What do I do now?"* I thought, feeling very 'labeled.' Without a backup plan, I knew I was at-risk for not getting the emergency care I needed in the future.

Recognizing this was an incomplete diagnosis, I feared for what was ahead for me. Worst of all, I knew that if I got sick and required ER medical care in the future, the new diagnosis would be confusing for the doctors there and could delay my getting much needed emergency medical treatment. Putting that thought aside, I decided to put it all in God's hands once again. Surely He would help me as He always had in the past!

Confusion in the ER

Just weeks after our phone conversation with Dr. Pinckney, I became acutely ill with complications from a respiratory infection after aspirating a pill. It was the weekend, and my primary care doctor was unavailable, so I called Dr. Pinckney's office to see what I should do.

No one responded to my call, so after waiting a few hours, I went to the local hospital ER. The triage nurse recognized I was having trouble walking, talking, and breathing, so she took me right into the back with no waiting.

Why are you here today, Mrs. Gill?" the nurse asked. *"I am winded and having trouble Breathing, speaking and walking."*

Had I still had the previous diagnosis, myasthenic syndrome, they would have understood what to do. But I did not as that had been rescinded and I was virtually undiagnosed yet again. At that point, we were back to calling the symptoms myasthenia-like syndrome again.

"What do you want us to do for you?" she asked.

"I am having trouble breathing and I think I need an antibiotic," I said with winded, garbled speech. By this point, they clearly seemed like they could not understand my speech, so my friend Linda who brought me spoke on my behalf.

"Who do you see for this muscle condition?" the doctor asked. *"We can't treat you here. Our plan is to move you out and send you down to University downtown."*

The nurse returned and said, *"The doctors here don't really want to treat you as they don't know what to do."* Then she left the room as I sat teary and speechless. Upon returning, she said, *"Dr. Pinckney wants to talk with you on the phone, Mrs. Gill."*

"Mrs. Gill, what do you want us to do here? We can bring you down to University, but I'm not sure what we would do for you."

"No, I don't want to go to University. I just want to go home," I said with labored, garbled speech, feeling like a bother. The ER doctor wrote me two scripts. One for Cipro, an antibiotic, and the other for a myasthenia drug called prostigmin and I returned home to my bipap breathingmachine.

Curious…They never even offered me oxygen at the ER, despite my having been winded for days. Later, after finishing the Cipro, I read that it can cause neuropathy, hence my increased difficulty walking. However, the antibiotic initially worked well, as did the prostigmin. As we had hoped, my breathing improved, my garbled speech cleared, and all was well after a few days, except for a few unwelcome side effects from the prostigmin: night terrors

& diarrhea, which washed out my depression medications, and required an unplanned visit to my psychiatrist to get the antidote! Sometimes the only way to look is up.

I prayed about what to do, and it occurred to me to try to return to my previous neurologist, as Dr. Pinckney seemed to have a research agenda for me that superseded my circumstances. I was most disappointed in the way that Dr. Pinckney had gotten my trust then in a sense, become indifferent and stepped away. Since my condition had improved beyond the wheelchair, I was able to return to my longtime neurologist. He welcomed me back and reinstated the myasthenia-like syndrome diagnosis, as a clear diagnosis was still elusive after 35 years.

Since returning to my neurologist I have had two more emergency room visits and spent five days hospitalized inpatient for exacerbations over the past nine months--and so the medical merry-go-round continues. However, during that time, we have discovered that IV Solumedrol steroid treatments are very helpful and effective in treating my condition. I now have an RN case manager with my insurance company who is helping me navigate the healthcare system so I will hopefully not continue to 'fall through the cracks.'

Though I still am only virtually diagnosed, I feel confident that my medical team will provide practical help to me to navigate the ups and downs, the ebb and flow of this condition, with God at the helm. In all this, I realized once again that God has a plan at every turn in my life. Yes, in prayer, the Lord had led me to Dr. Pinckney, and to his credit, he helped me get out of the wheelchair and to begin an exercise program. But it seems God's plan did not include my staying under his care beyond three visits. In my heart and mind I knew that returning to my former, longtime neurologist was the best thing to do for my physical health and my peace of mind.

Flexibility is vitally important when placing your challenges under God's loving care!

SILVER LINING

I have learned that beyond the mind-body disconnect, there stands yet two other factors that affect physical, mental and mental health issues in the most amazing ways: faith and prayer. I have also personally found that by adding fervent prayer and Bible reading to my daily routine, I have been able to realize some focused healing in body, mind and spirit. This is what I call, *The Mind-Body-Faith Phenomenon©*.

The doctors may not always know what to do for me, as I remain virtually undiagnosed, but Jesus is ever present, twenty four seven. Prayer requests require no waiting rooms, no office hours, and God is ever present and omniscient. I believe that medical science is a trial and error art form that needs perfecting. In prayer, however, no matter how down or sick I feel, I can grow in gratitude and praise to God and affirm, again and again, that God is in charge of my life. Left to my own devices, my life is very different. In my humanness, I need to work hard to be dependent on Jesus for all my needs throughout my day to keep me fully on track with myself and others.

Sometimes it is hard to believe that Jesus is as present in our lives as He is. Yet I have personally benefited from having Him by my side at every turn in the road. I, for one, believe! I have found that in times of adversity, I am more likely to turn to God for help with little things and big things. This pattern of dependency on Jesus and the Holy Spirit started early on in my youth.

When I am believing, and trusting in God, I am more able to turn to Him for help and to ask Him to sustain me. However, I am more apt to try to go it alone when all is well.

For me, going it alone is all about self-sufficiency, trial and error. It sounds good in theory, but for me, going it alone, without Jesus, is unsustainable. For in as much as I believe that God has a plan for my life, I need his love and discernment, protection and comfort, His healing power in my life, desperately. In my mind, it is an illusion to think that I can do this life without God's help.

In my youth, I turned to Jesus, my Protector and Savior, The

Great Healer. During times when I have been unable to pray for myself, I have benefitted mightily from the coveted prayers of many praying friends and family. For what better help could anyone have than to invite Jesus, the Savior, Great Healer and Almighty Comforter, to be at their side through prayer???

Truly, sometimes along my journey I have been so low, there is only one way to look, and that is up. And that is exactly what I have done over and again in the face of life challenges. I have leaned heavily on my lifelong Catholic Christian roots to spiritually and emotionally sustain me, and return me back to a point of resilience, peace and joy as I revel in Jesus' presence in my life.

For me, great things really do happen when faith and prayer are added to the mind-body connection. In fact, it becomes what I call, *the Mind-Body-Faith Phenomenon©*!

For me, this concept is all about belief and trust in God, something that has challenged me my entire life. It is about steadfastly praying for whatever you need and believing that God will show up and make all things new. Moreover, it is about growing in gratitude for all that God has done and is doing in my life.

I have grown to recognize that all that I am, all that I do, all that I have, belongs to the Triune God, the Creator, and Savior through the power of the Holy Spirit. Obstacles relating to infirmity and disability seem to pale when compared to Jesus' peace, power and majesty.

I have learned to live by faith, rather than by sight, to embrace what comes with greater fervor, and let go of what I no longer need without regret. Most of all, I have learned to put aside my own pride and perfectionism and to appreciate the power of God's forgiveness in my life. That is, the power to forgive and the power to accept forgiveness.

In as much as Romans tells us that *"ALL THINGS work for good for those who love God,"* experiencing deep, major depression in 2007, as hard as it was, was paradoxically both a horrendous torment and a great blessing for me all at the same time. It was the beginning of healing my early life trauma from the inside out, and the start of my new life in Jesus Christ!

The absolute reality is that the mind and body are very closely connected, with shared chemistry, and psychiatric care IS an important part of mind-body care whether it is perceived that way or not by professionals. After all, psychiatrists are medical doctors. This forced separation is harmful to patients in part because of the stigma that goes with depression and mental illness, and only propels patients to avoid getting the care they sorely need. Looking forward, I see an urgent need for more collaboration between the medical field and psychiatry. As a patient, it has been confusing and disheartening to see the gaping exclusivity and territoriality between these two areas of health care.

Looking back, in the face of fear and angst about what was to come health-wise, I realized early on that any optimism I could muster would go a long way in helping me and my family cope with each passing day. In that way, one day, I made a life-giving decision about how to deal with what was transpiring. In the spirit of 'Bright Eyes,' and reminiscent of how I coped in childhood, I decided to seek peace and joy in Jesus and depend as fully as possible on God, while embracing optimism and trusting in Jesus. Doing this is a *conscious daily decision*, one that is at the heart of my healing process. It was not an easy decision, as it would take trusting in God with all my heart. This optimistic decision has led me to be able to be more upbeat, even joy-filled, despite adversity, and to pray daily, asking for whatever I need, even small things. I turn to Jesus in prayer with whatever I am concerned about. I also read Holy Scripture each day when possible, and am growing in gratitude for all my many blessings and challenges. This is the great transformation that accompanies *The Mind-Body-Faith Phenomenon©*.

I am fully confident in my soul that Jesus is always with me, I am not alone. He has a plan for me and my life, and I trust that He is absolutely capable of, and prepared to, provide a blessed good healing for me. Though I don't know exactly how or when He will accomplish this good work in my life, I believe and trust in faith that He will! I believe praise and gratitude to God are the keys to great blessings of peace and joy! These days, He is my strength, the one I turn to when I am feeling low, when all seems lost, and despair and feelings of hopelessness begin to roll in. Though I have experienced despair numerous times in my life, I have come to see it as both a spiritual issue, as well as, an emotional one.

For me, in calmer, less emotional times, I have come to think of despair as a sign I am not trusting God enough, forgetting that He is in control—not me. Unfortunately, it is a great temptation for me to pull away from people and situations when I am anxious, sad, or stressed.

To 'check out,' if you will, and step away from trying to deal with life on its terms. Generally, these days, when I find myself slipping into sadness and angst about my health, I try my level best to pray and refocus on what is most important. Best of all, I have praying friends and family that I can and do ask for prayer when times seem bleak or overwhelming.

To stoke optimism and faith, I have strategically placed some calming, Holy Scripture around my home in places I frequent such as my kitchen, office, and bedroom. Some of the passages read as follows:

"The joy of the Lord is your strength."

Nehemiah 8:10

"The Lord is my strength and my shield; my heart trusts in Him and He helps me."

Psalm 28:7

"Commit your way to the Lord; trust that He will act."

Psalm 37:5

"All things work for good for those who love God."

Romans 8:28

Faith, optimism and attitude adjustments have been very important focuses in maximizing my health and well-being since my tumultuous youth. I believe that optimism is the reason why I am still able to coexist with this most unwelcome mind-body disease while living a full life with close friends and a loving family, and I have been managing this for well over three decades.

Yet my neurologists have told me they have been treating me with palliative care for years, and they expect this degenerative disease to progress.

With that knowledge, I have, at times, had reason to entertain giving into despair as the depression, PTSD, and neuro-immune condition are so far reaching and all encompassing. I certainly have done that in the past. Yet, when I place my trust in Jesus, without taking it back as we all sometimes do, I have found uncommon strength, peace, and contagious joy, even in adversity, because of Him. He carries me on His shoulders through stormy waters. He wraps His arms around me to comfort me. Shoulder to shoulder, Jesus walks with me in His ways so I am able to rise above despair simply through the utterance of His holy name.

That optimistic decision was to pray, trust God and believe that He would heal me in His own special time and way. Trusting in God, my husband, family and caring friends, I pray often, and I have been trying to go about my life focusing on Jesus, and staying busy, especially through ministry, as much as possible. I continue to do things with my family, go to Sunday Mass, am active in prayer team at church, serve weekly at the local soup kitchen as a chaplain, participate in ministry outreach, serve on the evangelization team at church, write books and 'The Inspiration Café' blog, write, paint, sew, and make cord rosaries for the missions.

The truth is, I have found that faith and belief in God's healing power are far greater than any medical treatment for me. Jesus can and will do the most amazing things in your life, and that of your loved ones, if you but ask Him as specifically as possible! I am learning that Jesus will pave the way, provide healing, comfort and protection–and save me from any circumstance, simply for the asking. He is there for all of us at every turn in a most personal way, and stands in wait with outstretched arms to welcome back all who have strayed. I find I just need to trust him with all my being, and that is exactly what I plan to continue doing--come what may. I believe in and leave plenty of room for miracles. I trust in God that one day, whether today, or in my later years, or at the end of my life, I WILL be healed! How do I know this? Because I am a believing Christian, and trust in God's grace for me in my life. I know that though that thought defies the logic of the [medical] world, I treasure the emotional respite I get--just from thinking about Jesus healing me in His own special time and way!

According to the online research article, <u>Modes of Hoping: Understanding hope and expectations in the context of a clinical trial of complementary and alternative medicine for chronic pain</u> by

Emery R Eaves, hope is also vitally important in the production of life-enhancing endorphins.

When I am steeped in optimism and prayer, I can feel my blood pressure go down, and experience calm and peace, as anxiety and depression fade. I feel emotional relief just thinking about the possibility that God can and will heal me one day. For that I have great gratitude to Him.

You see, I have learned that every day is a new adventure, but I am confident that Jesus Christ is with me on this challenging journey. I believe I am never ever alone, unless I walk away from Him, as Jesus is by my side through the power of the Holy Spirit. I trust in Him and His power to heal and make all things new prevails in my soul.

CHAPTER 9:
Silent No More, Victim No More

Thus says the Lord:

"For I know well the plans I have in mind for you,
plans for your welfare and not for woe, so as to give you a future of hope.
When you call me, and come and pray to me, I will listen to you.
When you look for me, you will find me.
Yes, when you seek me with all your heart,
I will let you find me, and I will change your lot."

Jeremiah 29:11-14 | New American Bible [NAB]

With Jesus at my side through prayer, awe-inspiring healing has occurred in my life, and is now in progress… I AM VICTIM NO MORE!!!…. Indeed, I am also SILENT NO MORE, as I am writing and sharing my story in the hope that I can help others who have experienced untreated trauma and mind-body illnesses to heal. Perhaps that could be you or a loved one.

Through putting aside my own medical issues to make room for helping others, I have found my life purpose in ministry. Today, my hope and trust are in full bloom as every day I place everything I have, everything I am, everything I do into the hands of Jesus Christ daily. My joy and peace have long been restored, and I have found my purpose in service to others. Ministry is the logical fit for me as I am still a caregiver at heart. But now rather than caring for physical bodies, I have transitioned into caring for the spiritual needs of others in need.

For many years after leaving nursing behind, I felt as if I had lost my purpose as a caregiver.

Hard to believe, but it took me about 25 years to finally let go of my desire to return to nursing.

But life has a way of coming full circle, and I eventually found my purpose again by 'reinventing myself' as they say in therapy.

Several months after getting discharged from the hospital in summer 2007, I realized I was feeling very alone in my plight. I felt as though my body and my mind had betrayed me, and once more I found myself very teary much of the time. I think it is fair to say that I am a weeper when I am depressed. I remember thinking, *"Why can't I just be healthy in body and mind like other people?"* I didn't know anyone who had been through what I'd been through, and felt lonely and alone. Then I reminded myself that everyone has a cross, a burden to carry. God made us that way by design.

Today, because of much prayer and medical treatment for the depression, my joy and zest for living has been restored. I have been able to give my life fully to Jesus Christ like never before. My greatest desire is to serve God, through Jesus Christ, to the best of my ability, with all my strength. Yes, I am still on the bipap respirator 12-14 hours per day. However, I am thrilled to be able to spend the 10-12 hours or so every day when I am NOT on the respirator writing blogs, books, and doing the ministry for the glory of God. I organize my day around the breathing treatments and rest from 2:00 pm to 4:30 pm each day, reserving weekday mornings for ministry, writing, and similar activities.

During remissions, I try to walk about a mile per day three to four days per week, alternating with rest, and am taking chair yoga. It is also in the morning that I write my blog, *The Inspiration Café*, and do ministry outreach. On Wednesdays, I volunteer at a Soup

Kitchen from 9:00 am to 1:30 pm, then dash home to get on my machine for a respiratory treatment. My days and rest periods are filled with prayer—for my own healing, and for the diverse intercessory prayer needs of many others living with cancer, poverty, grief, and physical and/or mental illness.

On days when I'm severely fatigued and breathing is difficult, I am grateful to God for the Bipap respirator that makes breathing so much easier as it provides mechanical ventilation. When my speech is garbled, I avoid the phone and use email instead while reminding myself that the setback is temporary. When walking becomes more difficult and I am very unsteady on my feet, I again, remind myself that this is just part of my human condition and just a temporary challenge. I know that my life has been simplified by being a believing Christian. Either I am here with friends and family serving God with all my being, or I am with Jesus for Eternity.

It is really just that simple!

As my childhood years evolved and merged into early adult life, I only grew in my love and appreciation for reading and sharing Holy Scripture. I consider reading the holy Bible pure joy, a quiet respite from the turbulent, chaotic life I have lived. But as time marched on in adulthood, I noticed that I became somewhat distracted by sadness and anxiety and riddled with memories and pressing questions about my childhood. Questions that I often felt I could not talk over with anyone. Who could possibly understand my past and where would I start?

My siblings seemed to have moved on, but in my mind, I had become stagnant for a time, as if mired in quicksand that threatened my very being, as the PTSD flash backs and nightmares refused to leave me alone for years. This persisted for decades, and I became aware that I had much work to do to get past the unforgiveness in my soul for the cruelty of my mentally ill mother and my father's unsavory underworld activities.

When the mind suppresses or represses experiences and associated negative feelings, it is a defense. It is my brain's way of attempting to protect itself. However, stuffing negative feelings can be very detrimental to one's mental, emotional, physical and spiritual being, as the body, mind and spirit are all connected through a shared chemistry. Every thought is connected to a mind-body chemical reaction, which, if one is on overload, can displace stress into the body, while dulling or numbing a person's memory and spirit. In that way, the mind, body and spirit are closely connected through shared experiences and natural biological chemistry.

When I experienced significant childhood trauma and it went untreated, it set me up to be a victim for life. But it didn't need to be that way, and that has been remedied. That mindset, even when it is subconscious, can predictably infiltrate and alter one's physical, mental, and emotional chemistry on a cellular level, causing illness in mind or body, or both, often through damaging the immune and neurological systems. In truth, there is a huge cost for remaining silent after childhood abuse/trauma as I did for decades. As I grow, heal and learn to embrace my past, live in the present, and begin to take baby steps toward the future, I am finding that I not only like who I am-I am now able to love myself, possibly for the first time.

Everyone has a cross, a thorn if you will, of some kind in this life. Everyone has something or someone difficult they have dealt with in the past or must deal with in the present. It is just the way life is. Once I was able to begin dealing with my own mind-body issues, I began to grow and move on to the greater purpose that God has prepared for me and my life.

In my case, my wounds were deep, embedded shrapnel and I needed prayer, a good therapist and medications to help me move from broken to blest. It was, at first, very hard to admit to myself and others that I needed help because of the way I was raised. I had to recognize that I had adopted my mother's phobia for psychiatry and anti-depression medications. In that way, I had inadvertently become averse to taking any kind of medications for depression.

For me, getting help required my finally opening the doors and windows to my greatest fear, and admitting I had depression. From all that had transpired in my family in my childhood, I was in dire need of someone to help me after being silent for so long. I needed someone to encourage me, and help me find myself and my life purpose. In and out of therapy for years, it was not until I was 49 that I hit my wall and really tried to seek help. Finally, I found an experienced and patient psycho-therapist, Karen, and a wonderful psychiatrist, Dr. Efim Weinman, to help me heal from untreated childhood trauma. I really think I waited so long because of fear and pride.

Fear, from having lived with my severely mentally ill mother, and fear I would be like her, and would have to go through what she went through living with physical and mental illness, and pride because I was afraid of the social stigma associated with depression, PTSD, and mental illness in general. In reality, therapy validated my pain and allowed me to heal and move on with my life.

As my neurologist once told me emphatically when I told him about having depression and PTSD from untreated childhood trauma: *"You have to get that junk out of there!!!"* This book started as my own catharsis, my own attempt to rid myself of the toxins of untreated childhood trauma that were haunting me. And to that end, I was quite successful in accomplishing that goal.

I have been able to *"Get the junk out of there,"* so to speak, and move on, at last!

For many people with PTSD, nightmares and flashbacks are common. So common, in fact, that they are recognized as hallmark symptoms experienced as a result of this disorder. In my case, I was so flooded with both that I only wrote them down if they were serial or repeated, that is, if I experienced them in both nightmares and flashbacks. My nightmares and flashbacks included long ago forgotten familiar people, localities, and events in my father's world that corroborated closely with other pieces of my life puzzle already recalled. For the most part, they brought many 'déjà vu moments' to mind as they filled in the missing puzzle pieces for me. However, not until I began writing it all down did it make any sense to me. The new memory pieces seemed to perfectly fit the longstanding memories I had retained. It was as if the Lord had shielded me from my own memories until the time was right and I was strong enough to face my youth and deal with the untreated childhood trauma.

I believe the greater the pain, the deeper the wound and the greater the need is to remove the thorn. Like a splinter long-embedded in an old wound, it is important to carefully, skillfully remove the thorn in order to begin the full healing process. For some, emotional thorns may be but a tiny splinter near the surface of the skin that is easily removed. Yet for others, like me, the healing might be likened to surgically removing gun shrapnel from a gaping wound.

In the case of untreated childhood trauma, it is important to consider the extent of the wound, the source, and obtain the necessary help to take proper care of it. Hopefully, once the embedded proverbial 'thorn' is recognized, it is possible to name it, claim it, and deal with it in the here and now, and move on with life. Sometimes it is important to get professional help to heal. In fact, for deep thorns, as in the case of untreated childhood trauma, it may be necessary. Through soaking prayer, medication and psychotherapy, I was able to get my life back. Soaking prayer occurs when there are two or more people praying intercessory prayers for an individual. These prayers are especially powerful as Jesus said, *"Wherever two or more gather together in prayer, Jesus is in their midst."*

If you believe your thorn is a deep wound, or something just doesn't feel right inside as you read this book, please consult a therapist who can help you. Don't wait until you hit the wall like I did, and are absolutely broken and unable to function in your daily life. It may be a sign that memories are starting to bubble up, and you may be ready to deal with something that happened to you in your childhood that went untreated. Pray, trust your gut reaction, and recognize this important fact: *You don't have to do this alone. Professional help is available, and Jesus is just a prayer away.* I was unaware of the full extent and depth of my hurt until I began to let it go and to heal and evolve. Sometimes I have had to step away from toxic people in my life, as I did my mother. I felt overwhelmed and was sorely challenged to deal with my own childhood hurts and early traumatic memories, and had little time or energy left over to nurture others.

Human in every way, your parents may have experienced mental illness like my mom, or other issues of their own. They may have had mounting financial challenges that left them feeling anxious, down-trodden, vulnerable, and drained, living in poverty with little money, and withlittle energy needed to care for you. They may have experienced addiction or medical mayhem in their lives living with poor or failing health right when you seemed to need them the most. Like my own parents, it is possible they also suffered from mind-body dysfunction, untreated mental health issues or complicated lives that caused them to be abusive or neglectful of you in your youth. Yes, it is possible. Any combination of life experiences is possible. But is any of that your fault? Absolutely not!

Though some families may have an easier time of it than others, each of us is so different, so unique, that we each have our very own baggage to deal with in this life. Certainly, we all have something we need to deal with in life. Some think that going back over untreatedchildhood trauma is a sign of weakness, but I believe, with all my heart, that it is the hallmark of a sound mind, courage, and strength. In my case, I had no choice but to seek help due to mind-body issues. If there is a childhood trauma holding you back in your life, try to deal with it head on, lest it negatively affect your mental, spiritual, and/or physical health, as well.

When I lay my burdens down in Jesus' hands, I have been amazed at what happens. I have reaped some of the greatest healing treasures, in body, mind, and spirit. By doing so, I have gained insight, peace, and even joy! God has given me rest for my ruminating mind as well as for my body. Additionally He infuses me with His holy Spirit which allows my soul to make it all happen and come together according to His plan! As Christians, I believe we have been offered the greatest invitation of all times. It is the same invitation given to your ancestors, and mine, and it is the same one in place for our children and for future generations!

*"Come to me, all you who are weary and burdened,
and I will give you rest."*

Matthew 11:28-30

In looking back over my life, especially, my traumatic childhood, *a place to visit but not to dwell,* some have told me the past is done, over, that it is time to move on. However, for people like me, things may not be quite that simple due to the mind-body connection presenting so many life-challenging complications.

> *"Let us hold fast to the hope which we have professed*
> *and never turn away from it.*
> *God has given his promise, and He can be trusted."*

Hebrews 10:23

There are so many places I have searched for hope within myself, other people, my doctors, and chance. But today, I place my trust and hope squarely in Jesus Christ, with the understanding that He will, indeed, "Work all things for good for those who love Him," my hope is now lasting and eternal. Sometimes in the past, I have placed my hope in things and other people, only to find that my hopes can be easily dashed and slip away. I know this all too well from my youth. But when I place my trust and hope in God, I can rest assured that He will work all things out for good as He has done for me all my life, repeatedly. This is a source of great joy and deep abiding peace for me.

I pray often and fervently with a sense of anticipation. I can hardly wait to see what God will do next in my life. Only God has the 'full picture,' the broad overview of every circumstance inanyone's life. Jesus is actually the reason for my hope. When I place my hope and trust in Him, He dependably works things out for good as he does for all of us. His promises are enduring, so there is no need to second guess the outcome of any situation. Hoping in God has allowed me to let go of my need to control every situation. He takes care of it all *despite* my unbridled worry and angst, and my propensity to 'take it back!'

I have found when I place my trust in The Lord, worry ceases, anxiety clears, and faith and optimism prevail. Only then am I able to walk in the confidence of knowing that God is the trustworthy steward of every prayer I utter. He will see me through, and work things out for the best, and for that I have peace of mind even in the face of extreme adversity.

I like to pray often throughout the day, but some days it takes all my strength to resist the temptation to despair and 'take back' the prayer-filled trust I place in the Lord. I believe thatthe Lord is trustworthy with my greatest concerns, and the deepest desires of my heart. Before I even utter my heartfelt prayers, He stands in wait to answer them. His answer may be yes, no, maybe, or not now, but I know I can be sure He will work things out for the best. Place your past, present and future—your hope--in Jesus this day, for He is the essence, the very source, the definition of hope eternal!

Some days, I look out my front window at the open, hilly field across the street from my home, and close my eyes imagining that I can run up the hill. Sometimes when it is snowing, I imagine that I can ski down that hill. I envision walking across the street and down the hill to visit the horse farm there in the valley by the tree-lined fence, or that I am flying a kite, or dancing, all things I have longed to be able to do.

Somehow, it seems I was born an optimist, and usually try to see the good in situations and other people, despite what is/was, which is why my parents called me 'Bright Eyes.' I think it was God's grace that helped me grow in confidence in what my mother told me about God, Jesus, Mary, and the Holy Spirit, and somehow they became the center of my being to endure both Mom's rants and wrath, and my father's world.

Though it appears I am on the 'Miracle Installment Plan,' I know I will be healed one day because I am a believing Christian. Even if it comes at the end of this life or in the next life, I have much to look forward to as a new creation in Jesus Christ! Jesus is far bigger than my fears, worries, and problems. Who else can be trusted to conquer evil and darkness in your life, heal your pain and illness, provide abundantly beyond all measure, and be the lover of your soul?

Most of all, who else has given his life in exchange for our sins?

> *"I am the light of the world.*
> *Whoever follows Me will never walk in darkness,*
> *but he will have the light of life."*

John 8:12

Every day I try to take a few minutes to pray for Jesus' help, *"Jesus, I trust in you."* I take a leap of faith, hope and trust that Jesus will help me this day in a multitude of ways. By so doing, I have nothing to lose, and everything to gain, as I step out of darkness into the Light. I so believe in this concept of trusting God, that I often wear a special religious Divine Mercy medal with a picture of Jesus on one side, and the words, "Jesus I trust in you" on the other side.

At times, fear can temporarily stop us in our tracks, and prevent us from moving forward in ourlives. It can disorient a person, turning the day into night, and provoke anxiety, depression, and despair, a "Dark Night of the Soul." In our humanity we were made to seek out light. Optimism is a personal choice we all can make each and every day.

Silver Lining

Yes, today, I am happy to be silent no more, and victim no more. The door to mind-body wholeness has been opened, and I can now see that my greatest blessings have come from my greatest hurts. It is hard to imagine my life without the abundant blessings that hope and faith bring. For with them, I can experience each day as a new adventure, rather than something to take for granted, tolerate, or even dread. Truly living a hope-filled life means that we understand the reason for our hope. Hope for success. Hope for wellness. Hope for financial security. Hope for inner peace. Sure, all these things are important; but I have found in my own life that there is no greater hope in this world, than Jesus Christ.

> *"Your greatest ministry will likely come out of your greatest hurt."*
>
> Rick Warren, author,
> "The Purpose Driven Life"

At times, I have been stormed and haunted by physical suffering, discomfort and hurt, as the result of depression and PTSD; other times by circumstances, such as medical issues, a traumatic childhood, homelessness, and the loss of a loved one. But in as much as 'suffering happens,' I have found that the Lord can harness times of extreme challenge for the common good. For example, when one who has a disabling illness is willing and able to empathetically help others in some way, despite the condition. Or possibly one who grieves the loss of a loved one can eventually muster the strength, through weakness, to reach out to others around them who have lost a loved one. In a way, that is the 'story behind the story' of my own life.

In my mind, a hurting soul is just steps away from being a helping soul. And to that end, a restored, renewed, rejuvenated soul is the very life-force behind effective ministry. Personal trials and tribulations are often the best teachers for ministry to others, preparing individuals to seek God in earnest and allowing them to become "wounded healers" for others over time.

When I first asked Jesus to come into my life I was probably about 6 years old. Shortly after, my mother and siblings were away during that dark period in my life, I felt absolutely alone as both of my parents were fully unavailable to me. Inviting Jesus in was like turning a light switch on in a dark room with no windows. Life seemed more in focus, less scary, and everything seemed clearer. I believe I became kinder and more able to see strengths and weaknesses in myself and in others, and grew to understand that there is strength in weakness, and weakness in strength. I came to understand early on that as a Christian, I am here to help other people in need. To that end, I have less need to be comfortable, as this life is merely the waiting room, a sort of dress rehearsal, for a life far greater than anyone can ever imagine.

Do not be anxious about anything, but in every situation, by prayer and petition, with thanksgiving, present your requests to God. And the peace of God, which transcends all understanding, will guard your hearts and your minds

in Christ Jesus. Philippians 4:6-7

Sometimes I find I get so busy with telling God what I want that I don't take the time to listen and wait for His answer, as I deluge Him with my prayer requests in rapid-fire succession. That pattern of communication has the potential to overwhelm anyone on the receiving end--even Jesus Himself. Rather, as in any conversation with another person, it is vitally important to take a deep breath, and look and listen carefully to the response of the one we are communicating with, as we share the peace and joy of Jesus Christ:

Finally, brothers and sisters, whatever is true, whatever is noble, whatever is right, whatever is pure, whatever is lovely, whatever is admirable–if anything is excellent or praiseworthy–think about such things.

Philippians 4:8

Some people say they never or rarely get answers to their prayers. I say it may be a matter of prayerfully taking the time to listen and watch and wait... For every prayer there is a response of some kind: Yes-no-maybe or not now. Prayer and reading the Bible are important avenues that alert us to God's answers to our prayers. What a tremendous blessing to have the Bible to lead us in discernment.

"Whatever you have learned or received or heard from me, or seen in me–put it into practice. And the God of peace will be with you."

Philippians 4:9

I like to pray fervently and often throughout the day for big things and little things, and I believe Jesus will hear and answer those prayers in His own special time and way. When I pray, I feel it is important to pray with confidence, knowing fully that my prayers do not fall on deaf ears. I believe that God hears and answers every prayer. He has placed Jesus at my side and yours to hear us and help us in everyday matters as well as when we are in great need. He is our compass and our light in this life.

I like to share my deepest burdens, hurts and daily life with Jesus throughout the day. I call on Him in the early morning hours when I rise, and at night when I am weary from a busy day, and I call on Him with prayer requests, petitions, praise and gratitude throughout the day. He is readily accessible beyond human imaginings, and stands ready to help us all reach for higher ground. To some, God may seem like a far-away deity, with a remote quality about Him. To others, He is seen as a relentless task-master, pushing them along in directions they prefer not to go. However, to me, God is a loving, heavenly Father, ever present, providing practical help, particularly in challenging times.

At times, it has been hard for me to fathom why Father God, Who spins the world on its axis, the Almighty Author of Life, would even consider having an individual, loving plan for me—as He does for each of us. But it is true! His plan is not for us to live in drudgery, despair, and woe, but rather, to have an abundant, peace-filled, joyful life in Him! Yes, there is a mind-body chemistry with my neuromuscular condition, depression and PTSD. And the times when all three exacerbations hit at the same time, it is daunting. Due to my medical issues, some days the temptation to despair, give up and give in looms large. But I have learned to fight these unwelcome temptations with all I have. Through prayer.

Despite enduring challenging health circumstances and issues, I am now convinced that God has a plan for my life. It involves volunteering in ministry with the homeless, the poor, the disabled, and the elderly. It involves witnessing to what I have seen of God in my lifetime. Every morning when I get up, I reassess what strength I have to work with for that day, and give God gratitude for being able to breathe, walk, talk and swallow. Breathing OK? Check. Speech? Check.

Swallowing? Check. Walking without falling? Check. Blurred vision? Check. Any day that I am able to breathe easily, walk and talk is considered a blessed good day.

The truth is, some days I am too sick to do ministry. It is those days that I designate as prayer days. Let's face it, it is hard to do ministry when you don't feel well. But many days I am able to help others and I do so with great joy. There are also days when I am dealing with depression and occasionally, despair. Some days it seems like a minefield just trying to get out of bed and stay out of my own way. But my heart is with the vulnerable and disenfranchised, so I take my medications, always leave an opening in my schedule to rest when I need to, and press on. Like so many people, I have come to believe that I am at my best when helping others, so that is my primary goal for each day. I am always looking for ministry opportunities to get involved in, and other ways to share Jesus with others.

I used to pray for an end to my health issues—body, mind and spirit. Now I pray for strength and healing in any and every aspect of my being. Over the last 35 years, I have grown to see God's hand in everything, as He strengthens me, prepares me, and comforts me anew each morning so that I can handle whatever comes with living day in and day out. In the spirit of "All things work for the good for those who love God," Romans 8:28, I am now finally able to praise God in all things, for daily victories and great blessings of abundant supply, as well as, for the daily trials that make me stronger with Jesus by my side.

Though I have been Roman Catholic my entire life, the major depression in 2007 eventually led me into a much deeper faith and a personal relationship with Jesus Christ than ever before. Up until that time, I thought I had strong faith. But I was humbled by the experience, and emerged much stronger! In actuality, once I accepted Jesus Christ into my heart in a personal way, I became far more ready to take on and share the fruits of the Holy Spirit with others. After doing so, through the power of the Holy Spirit, I became more prepared and equipped to be empathetic to others, more loving, joy-filled, peaceful, persevering, kinder, faithful, gentle and self-controlled as I become a new creation in Jesus. Hatred, and unforgiveness faded away, and the Lord replaced them with a kind and gentle spirit. It was a process, but one that led to a deeper understanding of the Mass, the Bible, and the Eucharist (Holy Communion).

---

*"Therefore, if anyone is in Christ, the **new creation** has come: The old has gone, the **new** is here!"*

2 Corinthians 5:17

When I began to seek The Lord with all my heart, eager to stand in His Light, I began to share in His peace and contagious joy. I soon learned that those who bow down before God in earnest prayer are comforted and receive healing in various forms. The joy of the Lord is not only contagious in all the best ways, it allows those who love the Lord to recognize each other, sometimes without ever speaking a word!

After my inpatient hospitalizations in 2007, I began to trust the Lord more and discover and embrace my very own God-given purpose. Over time, things seemed to just fall into place and there was a simplicity that resonated in my being. I recognized I had been truly broken, then healed, in body mind and spirit. The healing consisted of lost dreams and self-loathing going by the wayside, and anger and disappointment over what had been lost seemed to evaporate into thin air as I began to walk in the light of Jesus with a grateful heart. Things that were out of reach for me seemed to lose their shine and their importance, as I had begun to embrace my new life that God had prepared for me.

Feeling more whole, more integrated, in body, mind and spirit, I was able to access and use my faith in practical, unprecedented ways to accomplish new things as I focused more and more on others, and less on my own symptoms and shortcomings. Having endured abject poverty, untreated childhood trauma, and infirmity, I began to see the needs and vulnerabilities of others in a clearer light, and they became more important than my own. Yes, I had experienced unspeakable childhood trauma and loss; but that was transformed as I learned to console others who were poor, homeless, grieving, traumatized, and in need. For me, with Jesus at my side, there is always a brighter horizon, always a reason to hope, always a silver lining. I finally understand that in the Lord, there is no darkness at all. Prayerfully growing in discernment, I thirst for life-giving direction that only the Holy Spirit can provide. Sometimes you just have to put some things of the past to rest to be able to embrace your healing and the plan God has for you and move forward.

"We wait in hope for the Lord; He is our help and our shield.
In Him our hearts rejoice, for we trust in His holy name.
May Your unfailing love rest upon us, O Lord,
even as we put our hope in You."

Psalm 33:20-22

To do my part, I needed to first recognize that the only thing I own in this world is my God-given free will. That's it…There are no entitlements to happiness, or material things, and every good thing I have comes from God. God is all that is good by definition. It is entirely up to me to make good choices, great and small in this life. Each life choice I make has the potential to bring me closer to the triune God--Father, Son and Holy Spirit, or further away.

Sure, I have experienced challenges and lots of surprises in this life, but somehow, when I consciously place my confidence in knowing that God is in charge of my life, it all seems to go so much smoother. Yes, there have been many bumps in the road, obstacles and hurdles to jump over, but by following God's will, through His Blessed Son, our Savior Jesus Christ, I have been able to endure great and greater things, and be of service to others, despite adversity that comes my way. Actually, I revel in the sublime knowing that I am never alone as long as I stay on the Divine pathway he has laid out before me.

SILVER LINING

God's love for you and me is like an open umbrella that provides protection and comfort. When we follow His commands, He has us covered. Step away from the Lord's path, and you are no longer under His umbrella and protection from the rain. In fact, we are drenched and on our own until we seek Him in earnest once again, and step back into His all-encompassing care. That is why I always try to pray with confidence in all things, with the quiet knowing that the Triune God hears my prayerful pleas and is on my side, paving the way for greater things to come.

Today, I believe that there isn't any situation that the Lord and I can't handle together.

CHAPTER 10:
Moving From Broken to Blest

"The joy of the Lord is your strength."

Nehemiah 8:10 (NIV) New International Version

7 Steps to Move From Broken to Blest

Step 1: Acknowledge Your Brokenness

Step 2: Invite Jesus to Come Into Your Life **Step 3:** Evict Negative Thoughts about Yourself and Others **Step 4:** Reach For Forgiveness: The Key to Health and Happiness **Step 5:** Accept Your Own Imperfections & Those of Others

Step 6: Learn to Look For Silver Linings in Adversity

Step 7: Embrace the Healing That Awaits You

Though there will be some overlap, each step in this process is vitally important to initiate before the next step. Forgiveness is at the hub of effectively being able to put aside childhood trauma.

Step 1
Acknowledge Your Brokenness

"The Lord is my shepherd, I shall not want.
He makes me lie down in green pastures,
He leads me beside quiet waters,
He restores my soul.
He guides me in paths of righteousness
for His name's sake."

Psalm 23:1-3

These days--most days--I have great peace and joy overflowing to share with family, friends and ministry. Yet, being human as anyone else, I also have times when I feel broken. For me, these times have come into my life while living my stormy childhood with my mentally ill mother, when I was molested in my youth by the unwelcome stranger, in tow with my father while he was 'doing business,' when I lost my chosen career to infirmity, when I was hospitalized with major depression, and associated PTSD from childhood trauma. Exacerbations of generalized muscle weakness have only complicated daily life. During these times of brokenness, it takes all my strength and resolve to put one foot in front of the other and press forward. I strive to rise above feelings of emotional brokenness, and the physical discomfort of living with a disability.

During these trying times, it is hard to see my blessings. It is during these times that I allow myself to sing the blues for up to three days, according to my '3 Day Rule.' After that, I can usually settle down, and settle into my circumstance by:

1. Reminding myself that there are so many others with far worse plights.
2. Deciding that my condition flare-ups are surely temporary. As

a Christian, I understand that the issues and problems of this life do not follow us into the after-life I believe in.

3. Remembering what my psychiatrist told me: Clinical depression accompanies my medical condition because the acetylcholine in both my muscles and brain is depleted causing a mind-body chemical imbalance.

4. Recognizing that I have no control over the chemical imbalance, except for taking my medication and working on my attitude.

5. Realizing that I have state of the art medications and equipment to use, such as my 3 wheel walker, wheelchair, and Bipap machine, which saves me many trips to the ER.

6. Reminding myself that God is in charge and all is well.

After 35 years of infirmity, I have learned not to take myself quite so seriously. In this way, the medical exacerbations I continue to experience 3-4 times per year are diminished in my mind with regular attitude adjustments, and I am better able to cope—which is not easy, but with God's help, necessary.

STEP 2:
ASK JESUS TO COME INTO YOUR LIFE

"Be anxious for nothing, but in everything by prayer and supplication, with thanksgiving, let your requests be made known to God. [7] *And the peace of God, which surpasses all comprehension, will guard your hearts, and your minds, in Christ Jesus."*

Philippians 4:6-7

"If God is for us, who can be against us?"

Romans 8:31

As a lifelong Catholic, I always thought I had strong faith--until I was hospitalized for depression in 2007, and my faith was sorely tested. I knew about God and Jesus and the Holy Spirit, but my prayer life seemed to have gone from a beautiful rose to a withered flower. God seemed so distant. I found much of that time that I could not easily pray for myself. It was actually hard, if not impossible. Everything seemed difficult to do, even the smallest tasks. I depended on prayers I had learned in my youth that my mother taught me. The Our Father and the Act of Contrition, Spontaneous prayer seemed impossible beyond, *"Heaven help me,"* and *"Jesus I trust in You."*

Fortunately, I knew well that God understood my weaknesses and frailty, and that He wasclosest during times of despair and travail. I worried I would never be well again. Worry is a negative trait, and I needed to gird my heart and mind against it with all my God-given strength. Who can possibly endure living today while re-living yesterday while pre-living tomorrow all at the same time? It is impossible, and the recipe for exhaustion and defeat or fatigue.

Not all days are created equal. Some days are harder and more challenging than others. The above Scripture is actually one of empathy, an invitation from Jesus himself to you and to me. It is an invitation to all of humanity that Jesus has extended for over some 2000 years to bring our burdens to Him. True today as it was when Jesus first spoke these words, He cordially invites us to lay down our heavy burdens and to follow Him.

In my own life, I generally find there is good reason to pray to God at every turn. This is something I learned around the age of

6 from my mother just before she went to the mental institution. This practice continues today as I am in the habit of praying in the morning, throughout the day, and at night before bed. I pray both when I am down and during times of joy and trials. I pray when I have a need, and sometimes just to say thank you. I believe that simply for the asking, Jesus is with me to help me carry my burdens, to mend relationships, to comfort me and my loved ones, and to protect me in every way. He is the remedy for depression and despair. Jesus will go before me and pave the way by softening and changing hearts and circumstances. He goes behind me to serve as my body guard in times of danger and trouble. He wraps His healing arms around me as He walks with me, side by side, to comfort me in my darkest valleys.

In a way, fear is a lack of hope, and moreover, a lack of faith and trust in the saving power of Jesus. For when you believe, with all your being, that *"All things work for good for those who love God,"* Romans 8:28, it is easier to follow this scripture from Philippians 4:6-7. When you understand that God sent His Only Son to live and die and rise in expiation for our sins so that we can live life-eternal, it somehow all comes together and makes sense.

Though hard to admit, it is always a fearful time for me when getting up in the morning, have difficulty breathing when off of my respirator machine, and I fall for no apparent reason. Or when having 'over done it,' and my speech becomes garbled from respiratory muscle fatigue.

The potential to experience fear at these times is huge, but after all these years, I know that faith and fear cannot exist, so I try to always choose faith daily over fear. Fear literally disappears and is replaced by peace when I ask for Jesus' help, and move from a state of mayhem to deep inner peace. In fact, just repeating Jesus' name brings me great peace and joy. I like to try to pray even before calling a friend to vent, thereby replacing worry with hope in prayer, while living one day at a time. The Lord has strong shoulders and can easily pave the way for life's greatest challenges.

> *"Consider it pure joy, my brothers and sisters,*
> *whenever you face trials of many kinds,*
> *because you know that the testing of your faith*
> *produces perseverance."*
>
> James 1:2-3

STEP 3:
PUT ASIDE ALL WORRY AND FEAR

EVICT NEGATIVE THOUGHTS ABOUT YOURSELF AND OTHERS

> *"For God did not give us a spirit of fear,*
> *but of power and of love and of a calm and well-balanced mind..."*
>
> 2 Timothy 1:7 / Amplified Bible

Like many people, sometimes I have intrusive negative thoughts that must be dealt with swiftly lest they contaminate my peacefulness. At times we all ruminate on thoughts that are upsetting or unwelcome. However, I have found that it is very important to deal directly with these thoughts, and swiftly, before they become overwhelming and threaten to reduce me to a state of fear, worry, depression, and even despair.

In my own life, in the past, before extensive therapy, I often experienced ruminating thoughts, particularly at night when all was quiet while trying to get to sleep. Not only was I uncomfortable with the seemingly endless rehash of old negative tapes, I didn't really know how to make these thoughts stop. Worse yet, I didn't know I could! I was a world class worrier with way too much negative thought material. Night after night, I would experience repeat renditions of my mother's late night rants. Hateful phrases echoed in my head from when my mother was psychotic in my youth. The negativity made it hard to turn off my thinking, hard to get to sleep, hard to stay asleep, and needless to say, I was exhausted when I got up in the morning.

The idea of evicting thoughts may sound unusual or even funny to you, but it is each individual's right and, moreover, privilege, to only entertain the thoughts they choose. Another metaphor for this can be seen in sweeping out cobwebs with a broom. There is no need to allow spiders to reside with you in your home when you can get rid of them easily with a sweeps of a broom. And so it goes with negative thinking and ruminating thoughts. You must remove negative thoughts *as they occur*, lest they persist and overwhelm you, derailing you from keeping your focus on Jesus. If you have trouble doing this on your own, then by all means, ask for Jesus' help and see how quickly your peace and joy return!

In my life, when the blues roll in, I try to praise God and pray for His presence, His comfort, and His protection. I always try to begin my prayers by praising and thanking God, and pray in the name of Jesus Christ.

"... We take captive every thought..."

2 Corinthians 10:5

Step 4:
Reach For Forgiveness:
The Key to Health and Happiness

*"If you forgive others their trespasses,
your heavenly Father will also forgive you."*

Matthew 6:14

In my case, I had to forgive to get on with my life, and put my physical health, back on track. I was fully at God's mercy as I asked for his help to show me the road to forgiveness. I did not know how, despite my great desire to do so. In essence, it was a God job if there ever was one.

Only the Lord can give you a compassionate heart for those who hurt you. Only He can enhance your ability to love the unlovable, and forgive the unforgiveable. Through the power of the Holy Spirit, Jesus himself has given me an attitude of gratitude in times of adversity to face great things, against all odds.

Jesus is the greatest hope, the greatest joy and peace, I have ever known. Perhaps it's time for you to take a closer look at Jesus and ask for His help in your life, too.

Personally, I do not believe we have to completely *forget* the offenses of another who has hurt us to be able to forgive them. Memory recall is just part and parcel of our humanness. However, I do believe if we can pray for the person who has hurt us, it is an act of faith and of forgiveness. I find whenever I am able to pray heartfelt prayers for a person I must forgive, the offense fades in my memory and I am able to see their hurt, and their need. It has been said that "hurt people hurt others," and it is true. When I look again at my parents childhoods, I can see their hurts and it makes forgiveness a lot easier for me. I know this in part because I rarely, if ever, completely walk away from or turn my back on those who hurt me the most. I tend to keep those who have hurt me close, but if need be, I simply step away for a while, stay out of the fray, and quietly pray for them. For me, the power of prayer is a deep mystery, but I am convinced it profoundly changes the hearts and lives of all involved for the good.

Ask God, through Jesus Christ, to forgive you for your own offenses and those of others, those offenses you are aware of, and those you are not. Clearly, praying for those who have hurt you is a tremendous act of love that goes far beyond the limitations of our own humanness, merging with the Divine. The best thing to do is to learn to forgive quickly before unforgiveness has a chance to take root, as the roots of un-forgiveness are, unfortunately, pervasive, deep and enduring. Surely you know someone who has been severely affected by their own lack of forgiveness. With smoldering anger, sadness, or even infirmity, they live each day in torment with little relief, and these negative emotions may easily affect both their physical and mental health. But there is some really good news in all of this.

For many years—decades, actually, I had what I called justifiable anger and indignation at the thought of my childhood. Not only could I not remember or embrace the extent of the childhood trauma that I endured, nor did I want to. I held on to repressed memories, despite the fact that they were detrimental to my overall health and well-being.

For years I wondered how and why the Lord could ever have allowed me to be born into the family I was born into. I was angry at my parents, angry at God, and full of self-pity that left me feeling like a victim for more years than I care to admit. Then it dawned on me one day while I was praying the Our Father:

> *"Forgive us our trespasses*
> *<u>as we forgive</u> those who trespass against us..."*

It was as if a light went on in my mind and heart, and I realized for the first time that we really are all sinners, and God forgives each of us to the extent that we forgive others. We all make mistakes; we are all prone to the sin, and dependent on forgiveness. Life just is what it is, and it is how we deal with the various adversities that come our way that makes all the difference.

What a concept! If I do not forgive others who have hurt me in the past, I will not be forgiven by God for my own transgressions. I knew the hurt and deep hatred in my heart had to go, but I had no idea how to make that happen. The day I acknowledged my own sinfulness was the beginning of my letting go of those I held personally accountable for my pain, as I realized I could not do it alone. I needed God's help--real help. My reaction to what had happened in my childhood was all wrong. Worst of all, it was eating away at me on every level--physically, mentally, emotionally and spiritually. Something had to change, and that was me.

Clearly, my unforgiveness had very deep roots, and this was a "God-job," if there ever was one.

So I began to pray for healing of memories, and for those who hurt me most in my youth. I decided to give my tormented childhood to God, the Great Healer and Comforter, and depend on His grace to help heal my deepest hurts, bind my gaping wounds, and mend my broken heart.

Today, I can see, and I believe with all my heart and soul, that God, in His Almighty mercy sheltered me from experiencing the full blunt force of poverty, abandonment, rejection, and abuse of every kind that I endured. Jesus protected me, and made His presence in my life known to me in so many blessed ways. I think it is noteworthy that traumatic memories from what occurred during my childhood, especially the abuse that transpired while being left in the care of my father and his associates, continue to be revealed to me, through prayer, PTSD nightmares, flashbacks, and various people in my adult life who knew him.

Much healing has taken place, though I continue to live with some PTSD and some occasional depression, as well as, chronic and acute medical issues. Despite it all, by the grace of God, for the glory of God, much healing has occurred, and *I no longer see myself as a victim.*

Though some of the memories linger, the intense anger and sadness has dissipated, and I am able and willing to pray often for those who hurt me most. I am no longer captive to the past.

With a new perspective, and many years of therapy behind me, I feel truly blest as I fully believe that God was present through all the trauma in my childhood, and in His infinite mercy, protected me, comforted me, and loved me through it all. During those most difficult years, I learned to trust that God was the one in my life who would never hurt me nor would He leave me. No matter what. That belief, and the love of Jesus, have been extremely healing for me in my adult life.

With the Lord as my Light, I have been able to figuratively pick up the shards of glass from my shattered, traumatic childhood, harness the pain and suffering for good, grow in forgiveness, and reach for lasting healing in body, mind and spirit. Jesus is the reason for my long lost, restored memories, and for much of the healing that has taken place. His timing and ways are always perfect.

The Perfect Prayer
Our Father / Book of Matthew 6:9

Our Father, Who art in Heaven, hallowed be Thy name; Thy Kingdom come, Thy will be done on earth as it is in Heaven. Give us this day our daily bread; and forgive us our trespasses as we forgive those who trespass against us; and lead us not into temptation, but deliver us from evil.

Amen

STEP 5:
ACCEPTING YOUR OWN IMPERFECTIONS & THOSE OF OTHERS

Growing up, I tried not to let anyone outside of our home know about my family life. In fact, I made a career out of ensuring that no one knew I was always hungry, had few clothes, or discovered about the abuses that took place within my family. I got so good at it, that I actually repressed memories of the torment.. So I put on my happy face, and avoided having close friends in my youth, for fear they would come visit and my family secrets would be uncovered. It was, indeed, a lonely time, as I had no one to turn to but the school nurse. In essence, I wanted people to only see my best side, for fear they would not understand, judge or reject me.

Perfectionism also prevailed in my early adulthood. I worked hard to be the best wife, the best nurse, and the best new mother. In reality, this was the point where things started falling apart and there was nothing I could do. The more I tried to be 'the best,' the sicker I got. Emotionally, I knew I was fighting a losing battle on every front, but my mind would not allow me to see the error of my ways. By the time I left work on disability after my daughter was born, my muscles were so weak that I could not even sit and hold a garden hose to water the potted plants on our porch. If you simply look around you, there are images everywhere of supposedly 'perfect people.' Hollywood's thinking has permeated our culture, and we see that fact on TV, in movies, in magazines, etc. The perfect sculpted body, the perfect career, the perfect family. Though it was simply not humanly possible.

The world will tell you that perfection is obtainable. Though we strive to be perfect like Jesus, that thinking sets us up for failure. *The truth is, we are a striving people, rather than a perfect people.* We all make mistakes and we all make bad choices at times. We all sin. No one is good and true and right all the time. Yet, we try to do our best each day, and that is all that the Lord expects of us.

For in the pursuit of wholeness, continuity in body, mind and spirit, it is vitally important to put aside the illusion of one's own perfection, and strive to be the best one can be in the eyes of God.

In the end, who else matters? The Bible tells us, 'If God is for us, who can be against us?' When I am able to adopt this perspective, there is no more need to compete with my fellow man (or woman) in an effort to 'one up' them. There is no more need to impress others or walk in shame before those you have deemed as competitors. In this way, I am enable to focus on serving God with my whole-heart and mind.

STEP 6:
LEARN TO LOOK FOR SILVER LININGS IN ADVERSITY

Worry, in particular, is such a waste of time. How many times have we all worried about things that never happened, things that never came to fruition? How many days have you spent in angst because you were unable or unwilling to look on the bright side while waiting for more information about something—medical test results, etc...? Follow these steps and you will soon begin reaping the benefits of putting fear, anxiety and worry aside. Simple as they may be, you will be on the way to retraining your brain to automatically, and courageously, look for the bright side in any and every circumstance. Putting aside all fear, anxiety and worry, you are then clearly prepared to pray for whatever you need in any situation.

1. Try to assess the situation in a positive light
2. Choose to adopt the positive perspective until you have more information
3. Remind yourself that nothing lasts forever
4. Say aloud: "It is what it is," and "This is just for now; it is only temporary."
5. Pray for whatever you need

Finding Your Very Own Silver Linings

In order to begin finding your own silver linings, take a minute to count your blessings today, beginning with God's presence in your life. Take a look at all the ways He has helped you, though undeservedly, through His Grace. Pray and ask for whatever you need--abundant supply, healing, comfort, protection, and as with any other relationship, try to remember to say "thank you" to God for all the blessings you receive. When challenges come, it is important to remember that God allows them, but doesn't necessarily cause them, for God uses trials and tribulations for our benefit, and He is ever-worthy of our praise!

Surely I would not be writing this book if not for my very own early brokenness and abundant blessings. For I too know the piercing agony of untreated childhood trauma, and have had to face the harsh reality of living with the remnants of lost dreams and the physical ramifications and mental anguish that often accompanies childhood trauma. I have lived with the night mares of a childhood gone awry, and for decades into my adult life have had to reassure myself often that those years have come and gone. As many adult children of trauma, I have little memory of those harrowing years until recently, yet live with their lingering effects.

Like many people, my childhood was hard, really hard, but I have since come to understand that I learned a lot during those early years, and it made me a stronger person in the long run. I probably would not have gone into nursing had I grown up in a different family, as I learned the importance of compassion firsthand. Without the childhood trauma, I would probably be less motivated and less persistent, less patient, and less compassionate toward others, as infirmity is quite a training ground for these traits. No doubt I would be less prepared to deal with my own bouts with persistent depression, as well as the neuro-immune disease I live with that has caused the progressive neuromuscular disease I have endured for 35 years. However, when looking for my own silver linings, traits such as compassion, uncommon strength, patience, tenacious persistence, and long-running endurance emerge to help me cope with the fallout of early childhood and adult infirmity. As these traits have slowly come to the forefront in my own life, I am filled with tremendous gratitude to God for sustaining me through such mayhem and turmoil in my early childhood. For where else could one's strength possibly come from, besides the unfailing, unconditional love of the Triune God? We all have silver linings, but sometimes it takes some introspective detective work, or even some professional psychotherapy, to uncover them for, and in, ourselves. Disappointment happens. And it is probably one of the most unwelcome feelings anyone can have. Missing a job opportunity, not getting what you had hoped for, experiencing the reoccurrence of a medical condition, feeling let down by people you care deeply about—these are some of the many causes of disappointment.

From victim to victorious, I revel in being on the road to a triumphant, God-filled life! For I believe that in every circumstance, in each challenge, there really are silver linings. I understand that in disappointment, you may get the chance to look at situations in a new way, learn new coping skills, and get yet another personal growth opportunity. Most of all, you may get the chance to embrace your faith in new and unprecedented ways, even being able to pray in difficult situations for others who have hurt you.

---

*"I will give you a new heart
and put a new spirit within you..."*

Ezekiel 36:26

STEP 7:
EMBRACE THE HEALING THAT AWAITS YOU

*"Delight yourself in the Lord,
and He will give you the desires of your heart."*

Psalm 37:4

On my journey, I have had to reach for healing and forgiveness. I have had to turn my life over to God so he could restore and rejuvenate my life. I can hardly imagine what would have happened had I not been willing to do so.

Today, I believe that God has healing waiting for all of us, but we need to embrace our humanness to access it. Everyone has a past, present and a future, and living in today is necessary to grow in gratitude for all our blessings. Yes, it seems that I am on the 'healing installment plan,' meaning that I have not yet received a full healing. However, with that said, I have experienced many levels of healing in my life. Healing of memories, healing of my victim attitude, healing of some of my symptoms, healing in mind, body and spirit. I have grown in confidence in God's healing power, and I look forward to what He will do next. To embrace the healing that awaited me, I found it important to understand that God is ultimately in control of my life. And I am truly grateful for that fact. Walking in hope, I know with all my being that I will be eventually be healed one day in God's time and special way.

SILVER LINING

Let's face it – as in the laws of physics, there is always going to be positive and negative in this life. But I have found that in every circumstance, there is predictably a silver lining. There is always a reason to hope! If you are not by nature an optimist, looking for the silver lining in every situation may seem a bit foolish, even, outlandish. But did you know that it is possible to train your mind to think this way automatically? With a little practice, you can learn to promptly reframe your thinking so that every scenario, every circumstance has a positive twist, a sunny side, so to speak.

Sometimes you just have to look a little bit closer to find your very own silver linings.

As we have seen in previous chapters, there are many positive physical and mental health reasons that support the practice of optimism. Looking on the 'bright side' can also enhance your mood, change your mind-body chemistry, save you from having a bad day, and even help you have a much needed attitude adjustment. Even if optimism is forced when first learning to reframe potentially negative experiences in your life, before long, finding the silver lining soon becomes second nature, and the health benefits are significant in both mind and body!

CHAPTER 11:
Time to Banish Negative Thinking

*"Be strong and take heart,
all you who hope in the Lord."*

Psalm 31:25

1. **Identify Negative Thoughts As They Occur**

   Whenever you experience negative thoughts, or experiences, name them and claim them as soon as you become aware of them. This will enable you to continue onto the next step in this vital process of dealing swiftly with negative thinking.

2. **Banish Negative Thinking**

   To isolate and banish negative thinking, it is imperative that you change your thought process.

   This is accomplished by figuratively changing the channel on your TV. It is a conscious decision that requires action on your part.

3. **Escort Negative Thoughts Out Promptly**

   Close your eyes and imagine that someone has entered your home who is not welcome. Now imagine yourself walking them to the door, evicting that person, and closing the door of your home firmly behind them. Evicting negative thoughts is very similar to that. You and you alone are in control of what you think and only you have the power to change the channel whenever needed.

4. Focus on Positive Imagery

When negative thoughts press in, close your eyes and choose to focus on something you either really enjoy, like to do, or a place you love to be. Many people go to their favorite beach in their mind when asked to do guided imagery. The object is to immerse yourself in positive thoughts that make you feel good. This can also change your mind-body chemistry, by releasing feel good endorphins that enable you to stay on a positive track.

5. Surround Yourself With Positive People

The company you keep has much to do with how you think and feel. Surrounding oneself with loving, caring, positive people is imperative for a happy, healthy life. In as much as birds of a feather really do flock together, choosing your friends carefully will reap many benefits for you and also for them. Negative people can bring you down, leave you feeling negative and burdened and change how you see the world. Conversely, a caring, loyal friend can be a true blessing, especially through times of great challenge and adversity.

6. Stay Busy

They say that busy hands are happy hands, and it is true. Being idle and alone for long periods of time is never a good idea, as we all need people, structure, purpose, and activity in our lives.

Volunteering to help other people, getting involved in your community, learning another language, bicycling, skiing, exercising, pursuing hobbies like writing, crafting, knitting, tapestry making, or scrapbooking are all great ways to maintain a happy, blest life. These activities can keep you healthy, stay sharp and focused, and enable you to move forward in your life. They also may serve as a distraction for you from worry, fear, and negativity, while promoting a sense of well-being.

7. 'Speak Life' into every circumstance and relationship

Rather than speaking negatively, we need to avoid speech that lowers our spirits and pushes us into a state of depression and ultimately, even despair. By avoiding negative speech and using positive speech instead, we are then free to confidently 'speak life' and hope into every circumstance as our perspective is seen through the eyes of faith. Medical research has proven that positive people have more fulfilling relationships and enjoy better physical and mental health than those who are negative. Negative speech is a direct route to negativity, and various forms of depression, and should be avoided at all costs. Clearly, the social, physical, mental, emotional and spiritual costs of negative speech are simply too high to pursue, and must be replaced with life-giving speech that promotes health in body, mind and spirit.

In 2007, in the throes of major depression, with nowhere else to turn, after laying my life in God's hands in desperation, I began to grow into a personal relationship with Jesus Christ. I began to trust Him even through the fog of despair. To do so, I had to learn to *walk by faith, not by sight*. Over time, I have come to believe that Jesus really is who He says He is in the Bible.

As He has showed up in my time of greatest need time and again, I can see Him actually moving me in my life, from broken to blest.

There was no other way that it could have happened, but through Jesus Christ. In 2007, as the fog of despair began to lift, I was eventually able to get on with my new life in Christ. But first I had to quell the negative thoughts that haunted me from my youth. In my adult life I have given my life to the Lord, written four books, worked with the local poor and homeless living in the woods. I lead the Prayer Team/Healing Team at a local soup kitchen, have become a community chaplain, and belong to the Prayer Team at my church. Though I had felt ready for my life to be over at age 49, I soon learned it was actually a new beginning for me in Jesus Christ!

> *"Come unto Me,*
> *all who are weary*
> *and I will give you rest..."*
>
> *Matthew 11:28*

As I adopted more of a biblical view of this world from reading Scripture, it got slowly easier to pray than to worry. For me, worry comes from having a knee jerk reactions to life's adversity and was replaced by prayer before beginning to worry. Worry is a waste of time that must be eradicated before allowing it to get a stronghold.

Praying into this new relationship with Jesus is a life-giving way that is life-changing, for the better. Once you give your life to God, you will still have challenges, and lots of them, but your perspective will be different. In fact, close communion with Jesus will lead you to conclude that He is the best and only hope this world has ever known!

CHAPTER 12:
Contentment:
I Have All That I Need

"I have learned the secret of being content in any and every situation... I can do all things through Him Who gives me strength."

Philippians 4:12-13

The Secret of Contentment

When I first chose to follow and serve the Lord more closely, I realized that He had provided everything I needed to live a good life and more. I knew my life would never be perfect as humanness is a state of imperfection. I knew Jesus does not fully heal all believers, nor does he take away all of our problems, but the impact He has had on my life is profound and undeniable. He had allowed me to endure great things and live with new, restored purpose. When I decided to follow and serve The Lord with all my heart and mind, I was already a lifelong Catholic and thought I knew Jesus. However, I began to see myself and the world differently than ever before. My attitude and perspective received a major boost when I began to put the Lord first in my life. Up until that point, I had lived 50 years *knowing* about Jesus. Now, I wanted to have a personal relationship with Him and to share Him with others like never before!

Before that time, as a Christian, I tried my best to always live my life focused on hope. Today, while ultimately anticipating hope-eternal with God in Heaven, I hunger and thirst for a personal relationship with Jesus, the greatest hope the world has ever known, and in that, I have not been disappointed.

"My sheep hear My voice, and I know them, and they follow Me. And I give them eternal life, and they shall never perish; neither shall anyone snatch them out of my hand."

John 10:27-28

For me, what used to seem like climbing mountains now seems more like hiking scenic, rolling hills. What used to seem logically impossible has become possible, because "all things are possible with God." When I walk with Jesus as my shepherd, I have no reason to wander away as all my needs are met through His abundant supply. I am never, ever alone because He is with me and though generally unspoken, the Lord's sheep also know their own, as they flock together. More specifically, I am now able to recognize a stranger if they follow the Lord, the Great Shepherd, by their kind heart and loving demeanor, clearly revealing the fruit of the Spirit within them.

> *"Be kind to one another, tender-hearted,
> forgiving each other, just as God in Christ has forgiven you."*
>
> Ephesians 4:31-32

Personally, I do not believe we have to completely forget the offenses of another who has hurt us to be able to forgive them. Memory recall is just part and parcel of our humanness. However, I do believe if we can pray for the other person it is an act of faith and a major step towards forgiveness. I find whenever I am able to pray heartfelt prayers for a person I must forgive, the offense usually vanishes through the power of prayer, on the wings of the Holy Spirit. I know this in part because I rarely, if ever, completely walk away from or turn my back on those who have hurt me the most. I simply step away for a while, out of the fray, and quietly pray for them.

For me, the power of prayer is a deep mystery, but I am convinced it profoundly changes the hearts and lives of all involved for the good.

> *"Cast your burden on The Lord, and He will support you;
> He will never allow the righteous to be shaken."*
>
> Psalm 55:22

I pray heartily, and ask for God's help, I instantly have the privilege of stepping back from my burdens, with the knowledge that He is in control and will support me in the most marvelous ways. Truly the power of prayer is far-reaching, far past anything that any human can fathom.

Through prayer, hearts can be softened, perspectives can change, and circumstances can and do change in the most amazing ways.

"Do not conform to the patterns of this world,
but be transformed by the renewing of your mind.
Then you will be able to test and approve
what God's Will is His good, pleasing and perfect will."

Romans 12:2

Silver Lining

Over the years, I have grown by leaps and bounds in the way of contentment, peace and joy. I am able to focus on the beautiful remissions I have rather than the exacerbations I experience. It's all about perspective. I no longer look at the 'half empty' cup, but celebrate and marvel in that the cup is filled at all. Yes, medication and therapy have been helpful in attaining this state. But the truth is that it is my strong Catholic Christian faith that brought me up from the harsh darkness of depression. I have learned to face and stand up to my own demons of untreated childhood trauma and the associated mind-body infirmity. I am able to put aside fear and being a victim by walking by faith rather than by sight. I have grown in compassion, and love, for myself and others, and most times can trust Jesus with complete abandon. My daily goal is to reach out to others; to go where the need is the greatest, wherever God sends me is where I want to be, and in that way, through Jesus, I have conquered hatred, un-forgiveness and darkness in my life. In the name of Jesus Christ I am free of the bondage of darkness once and for all, and now I know that *I can do all things through Him who gives me strength.* Jesus is my light, my life and my rock, and contentment, peace and joy are mine.

CHAPTER 13:
~ Gratitude, Peace & Joy ~
Blessings Galore!

"May the God of hope fill you with all joy and peace as you [place your] trust in Him!"

Romans 15:13

Early on, in my youth, I realized that my best hope in this life rested in God. Actually, in all the turbulence and chaos of my family, there really was no one else I could depend on, no one to turn to. To this day, though I am happily married, have 2 children, and a wonderful family and good friends, I can tell you I still turn to Jesus in prayer throughout the day for things great and small. My heart leaps for joy at just knowing that Jesus is there for me through thick and thin; something I rarely take for granted. I am eager to share Him with others, especially through the writing of this book and posts on my blog, *The Inspiration Café Blog*. In my youth trust was a rare commodity, and something that I did not easily place in myself or others.

Sometimes I wanted to trust others so much that I often trusted people who were not trustworthy.

Other times, trust was an elusive butterfly, something I could not part with. As is often the case with adult children of trauma, trust issues are most prevalent when you grow up in a dysfunctional, uncertain, toxic environment. Especially in my middle school and high school years, I found that my faith in the Triune God—Father, Son and Holy Spirit-- was the only certainty that I knew in those difficult growing up years. And that in actuality, God was my real father, not Howie. Over time, I have been able to grow in trust of others by first trusting in Almighty God, my Creator, in Jesus Christ, my Savior, and then Blessed Mother, who seemed to be the polar opposite of my own mom. It was through the CYO youth program at our church and going to Mass at our local Catholic Church that I slowly learned to trust other people by observing in them the fruit of the Spirit, especially love, joy, peace, kindness, patience, persistence and faithfulness.

I grew to trust others by looking for these traits in other people before letting them into my world. Sure, some people say they are believing Christians, but their behavior tells a different story. Believing Christians are different as they are guided by their beliefs and most read the Bible and apply what they learn there. They are not perfect, but they are a striving people.

Certainly no one is all good or all bad, but I have deemed trustworthy those who consistently reveal the fruit of the Holy Spirit in their daily lives,. Actually, the fruit of the Spirit comes into one's life as a gift of receiving the Holy Spirit of Jesus. Like the song says, *'You will know they are Christian by their love, by their love, you will know they are Christians by their love.'*

Since the early days of my faith experience at St Camillus Catholic Church, I have concluded that Jesus is the greatest hope I have ever known. For me, He is the only hope, and I trust Him with all of my being, body, mind, and spirit. Almighty Savior, Prince of Peace, Healer, Counselor, Comforter, Protector, and Friend--Jesus is there for all who call upon Him in earnest. The Bible tells us that if you seek Him, you will find Him. And it is true.

> *"Ask and you shall receive, seek and you will find;
> knock and the door will be opened to you..."*
>
> Luke 11:9

Jesus will go before you to change hearts, remove obstacles, open doors and pave the way, basically do whatever it takes for you. He goes behind you to heal relationships and protect you from all harm. He walks beside you to comfort and console you in your every time of need. I can only imagine what my early life, my childhood, would have been without Jesus' saving hand. He has brought peace, and holy love into my life like no other. He has helped me reframe my childhood and harness childhood trauma for good, and to grow to become a seasoned, compassionate listener, with a love for ministry, and a passion for working with the sick, the poor, and the homeless. Jesus is the source of my joy, the kind of simple joy that comes from praying to God, through Jesus Christ, and reading Scripture daily. In that joy it is revealed that God is my strength – the very source of every blessing and goodness in my life. It is the realization that I no longer walk alone or carry a lifetime of challenges and burdens on my own shoulders, but I am able to lay it all before The Lord, and in His kindness, compassion and mercy, He will help me along the way.

> *"The joy of the Lord is your strength"*
>
> Nehemiah 8:10 NIV

Since deciding to follow Jesus Christ as my personal Savior, my life has changed in so many joy-filled ways through the power of the Holy Spirit. In fact, I have experienced an ongoing 'attitude adjustment' on many different levels. For me, this is the outcome of true and lasting healing from the inside out. I have learned much about myself and my strengths and vulnerabilities, as well as, those of others. Most of all, I have learned that there is strength in weakness, and I have new purpose in life. I now know where my strength comes from, and that joy in adversity is my gift to share with others. I have eagerly dedicated my life to sharing the unconditional love of God with others daily in word and deed. Truly, depending on God for all my needs has been a life-changing, joy infused experience, one that has propelled the writing of this book. For what good is a God-given blessing, if you only keep it to yourself?

As the years have progressed, I have decided that I want to serve the Lord with whatever strength I have. Since every new day is a new adventure, I am able to put aside all the 'shoulds'— 'I should be able to speak clearly without intermittent, garbled speech, 'I should be able to walk unassisted without a cane or walker,' 'I should be able to keep up with my children, family, and friends.' Instead, I am dedicated to using whatever energy I have for the glory of God. In return, by doing so, I have benefited from much healing, inside and out, experiencing peace, and joy. I have realized so many blessings for myself and my family. *Inspiration has replaced aspiration,* as I no longer hunger and thirst to return to nursing, but rather, have embraced my new life in ministry by working to emotionally and spiritually help those in most need among us. This change in life direction has been such a blessing. I experience new confidence in my faith life as a believing Christian, and embrace a new sense of purpose in my own heart and mind.

Long gone is the grief I used to feel after the loss of my career due to mind-body disability.

Living with depression, PTSD, and a neuro-immune condition has freed me to have more understanding and compassionate for others; to take the time to listen to and encourage others in their times of need to reach out to them with greater empathy in new ways.

Recognizing that God has a new plan for me and my life, while moving past the situational grief that often accompanies living with a serious disability, and wading through untreated childhood trauma, my life is a new creation in Jesus. My life focus is no longer on every symptom I experience in a day's time. Rather, I have chosen to embrace my uniqueness, and engage as fully as possible in my God given life's work in ministry. Had I continued to be able to stay on the professional path I had chosen for myself after college, I would be a seasoned registered nurse by now, preparing for retirement. I don't believe God caused this condition, rather I believe He allowed it. I accept that God had a different plan for me and my life, and I am excited to see what He will do next.

"The joy of the Lord is your strength."

Nehemiah 8:10

As a life-long Christian, wife and mother of two grown children, I have come to believe that simplicity is most helpful and necessary in the pursuit of Christian faith. Basically, when I understand that God loves me unconditionally, and I try to love and serve God with all my being, I can rest in the quiet knowing that God is with me. When you trust fully in Jesus, you have no need for worry, as peace takes root in your soul. You pray with confidence for whatever you need, and leave the details to Him to control what is both within and beyond your reach. With Jesus, I have been able to endure life-changing infirmity, and prevail against all odds. Without being shaken to my core. I can rise above it all as I am comforted by the presence of The Lord in my life, and am now able to quell fear and anxiety as they arise. Despite my traumatic childhood, I have at last found healing, peace and joy, and have a deep trust and confidence—the kind that comes with close communion with Jesus Christ, and for that I am eternally grateful!

Yes, like many others, my early life was filled with turmoil and chaos, poverty, abuse and untreated trauma, disappointment, anger, despair, infirmity, and abundant fear. But the Lord rescued me from my humble beginnings, from living a life of absolute mayhem. He saved me from a life of spiraling infirmity, in body, mind, and spirit, and lifted me up on eagle's wings, transporting me to a far more peaceful, joy-filled life in Him. He calmed the turbulent waters of my memories, and bathed me in His magnificent light. He surrounded me with other devoted fellow believers, and led me into a beautiful life with a loving husband, 2 beautiful children, and has taken care of my every need through blessings galore. My God is a living God who is most involved in my life; one who cares for me in every way. And I am eternally grateful for His divine presence in my life, manifested through gratitude, peace and joy each and every day.

Life is full of challenges, surprises, and blessings, and I have learned that I need to make the most of whatever comes my way.

Epilogue

In the spirit of 'silent no more, victim no more,' the writing of this book has been a wonderful avenue for catharsis and healing for me in mind, body and spirit. I am free now to tell my story with complete abandon knowing that God is in control of my life. With the help of a good health care team, I no longer suffer from living in the throes of major depression, PTSD flashbacks and nightmares. Through their tireless efforts to help me, I have been able to recover and embrace lost memories, have moved forward in forgiveness, and have reframed my early memories in a way that has melted away the devastating, stinging effects of childhood trauma.

This, in turn, has allowed me to help others find hope through the adversity they have lived. I have been able to put behind me the angst, fear and low-self-esteem I once knew so well.

It is my expressed hope that my readers, especially those who live with depression and/or PTSD and any sort of untreated childhood trauma, will find kinship and solace in reading my story, and become emboldened to check out The Healing Workshop in this book and seek professional mind-body health care as needed for themselves. How different my adult life would have been had I been willing to seek out help much earlier for my depression and PTSD! But that is water under the bridge now.

Most of all, I pray that my readers will grow in their ability to speak life into every situation they endure, embrace their own truths with fervor, and seek God's help daily through prayer.

Moving forward, I can only see blue skies and rays of sun light through storm clouds as I look diligently for silver linings, and pray I can help others to do the same.

There is a Catholic prayer that I first read in my youth that I think speaks volumes about choosing to live a blessed life. It is the Prayer of St. Francis. Here is the prayer I think says it all:

Prayer of St Francis

"Lord, make me an instrument of your peace...
Where there is hatred, let me sow love;
"Where there is injury, pardon; where there is discord, union
Where there is doubt, faith;"
"Where there is despair, hope; where there is darkness light; where there is sadness, joy."
"Grant that we may not so much seek to be consoled as to console; to be understood as to understand; to be loved, as to love."
"For it is in giving that we receive; it is in pardoning that we are pardoned;
And it is in dying that we are born to Eternal Life."

IF MY STORY HAS RESONATED WITH YOU AND YOUR OWN LIFE, PLEASE CONSIDER CONTINUING ON TO
PART II, THE HEALING WORKSHOP

Part II:
The Healing Workshop

The Healing Workshop is written for individuals and small groups in need of healing. From the *"Are you an Adult Child of Trauma,"* to the *"Healing Journal Workshop,"* this workbook section is designed to help the reader get in touch with their feelings and to begin to heal from any childhood or other trauma that may have occurred over time.

This Workshop is <u>not</u> meant to replace therapy in any way, but rather, to help the participant gain important insight into their life to experience healing. It can be used alone, or in a support group setting with 10 or less participants, or with a therapist to help those who have experienced various types of trauma in their lives.

If these questions resonate with you and bring up any painful memories, it may be helpful to see a therapist to help you on along on your journey. The format of The Healing Workshop to encourage individuals and support group participants to either read alone or discuss together. It may also be used as an adjunct together with a licensed counselor or psychotherapist.

Exercise #1 The Healing Workshop: Chapter Discussion Questions

CHAPTER 1 QUESTIONS
EVERYONE HAS A PAST, A PRESENT AND A FUTURE— NO ONE IS EXEMPT!

"I have appeared to you to appoint you as a servant and as a witness of what you have seen and will see of Me."

Acts 26:16

1. Where do you fall in the birth order of your family, and how would you describe your family of origin?

_____

_____

_____

_____

_____

_____

_____

2. Which do you focus on more—The past, present or future? Please explain:

___

3. Is there a time in your life you can remember that was particularly happy and care-free? Please describe:

___

4. Can you remember a time in your past that was particularly sad or challenging? Please explain:

_____

_____

_____

_____

_____

_____

_____

_____

5. In as much as the past is a place to visit, not to dwell, do you feel like you are able to live fully in the present?

   Yes   No   If no, please explain:

_____

_____

_____

_____

_____

_____

_____

_____

6. Do you feel at peace with your past, or do you find yourself going back over difficult parts of it in your thoughts and dreams, flashbacks and/or nightmares? Please explain:

_____

_____

_____

_____

_____

_____

_____

7. Do you feel God's presence in your life? If so, please describe:

_____

_____

_____

_____

_____

_____

_____

8. What does it mean to give witness to what you have seen of God? Please explain:

_____

_____

_____

_____

_____

_____

_____

9. Everyone has a unique way to <u>serve</u> God. How do you serve Him in your daily life?

_____

_____

_____

_____

_____

_____

_____

10. There are many ways to give witness to the love of God. How do you personally witness to others of what you have seen and experienced of God? Please describe:

_____
_____
_____
_____
_____
_____
_____

11. List 3 additional ways that you can give <u>witness</u> and glory to God in your life?

_____
_____
_____
_____
_____
_____
_____

12. All of us at times step out of our comfort zones for various reasons. Is there a type of service for God within your comfort zone that you enjoy?

_____

_____

_____

_____

_____

_____

_____

_____

Chapter 2 Questions
Birds of a Feather Really Do Flock Together

"I can do all things through Christ who gives me strength."

Philippians 4:11-13 / NIV

1. In one word, describe your family of origin:

_____

_____

_____

_____

_____

_____

_____

2. Every person is unique, as is every family. In a paragraph, please describe your family of origin:

_____

_____

_____

_____

_____

_____

_____

3. Birth order sometimes defines one's role in a family by age. What place did you hold in your family (oldest, middle, youngest, etc…), and were you comfortable with your placement? Yes   No   Please explain:

_____

_____

_____

_____

_____

_____

_____

4. If you had describe your family of origin in a word, what would it be?

_____

_____

_____

_____

_____

_____

_____

5. In one word, describe yourself as a child:

_____

_____

_____

_____

_____

_____

_____

6. Have you ever experienced hopelessness in your life? Yes   No   Please describe:

_____

_____

_____

_____

_____

_____

7. Prayer promotes healing in both the forgiver and the forgiven. Are you able to pray for those who have hurt you? If not, why?

_____

_____

_____

_____

_____

_____

8. How do you pray for those who have hurt you? Please describe:

_____
_____
_____
_____
_____
_____
_____

9. Where does your strength come from? Please explain:

_____
_____
_____
_____
_____
_____
_____

10. Have you ever been in a relationship that was not good for you? Please describe:

_____

_____

_____

_____

_____

_____

_____

11. How did you handle that relationship?

_____

_____

_____

_____

_____

_____

_____

12. What is the reason for your hope?

_____

_____

_____

_____

_____

_____

_____

Chapter 3 Questions
The "At-Risk" Child

"God, grant me the serenity to accept the things I cannot change..."

Reinhold Neibuhr

1. The Serenity Prayer is best known for its use in Alcoholic Anonymous programs or AA programs. How can you apply this prayer to your own life?

_____

_____

_____

_____

_____

_____

_____

_____

2. Would you say your childhood family was supportive, unified, and loving, or dysfunctional with disharmony? Describe your own family growing up:

_____

_____

_____

_____

_____

_____

_____

3. Have you ever, in your childhood or adult life felt truly alone? Yes   No   If so, how did you handle it?

_____

_____

_____

_____

_____

_____

_____

4. Were you ever called or considered the "Black sheep" in your childhood family? Yes   No   If yes, please describe:

_____

_____

_____

_____

_____

_____

_____

5. Did you have learning problems in your youth? Yes   No

   Please describe and discuss how these they impacted you:

_____

_____

_____

_____

_____

_____

_____

6. Do you feel close to your family of origin? Yes   No   Please explain either way:

_____

_____

_____

_____

_____

_____

_____

7. Did you ever have an 'event' or person in your life that made you feel "less than?"

_____

_____

_____

_____

_____

_____

_____

_____

8. Did you report this "event" to anyone at the time?

9. What was their reaction and were they able to help you?

10. Has this 'event' been a source of anxiety for you as time goes on? Yes   No   Please describe:

_____

_____

_____

_____

_____

_____

_____

11. How did you deal with that situation or person when you felt minimized or bad about yourself?

_____

_____

_____

_____

_____

_____

_____

_____

12. When we choose to live in today, we commit to dealing with life one day at a time. How do you live one day at a time without borrowing worry from the future?

_____
_____
_____
_____
_____
_____
_____

13. Are you prone to worry? If so, how do you turn it off to live in the present rather than the future?

_____
_____
_____
_____
_____
_____
_____

14. Do you believe God is ultimately in control or do you try to control everything in your life yourself?

Chapter 4 Questions
Naming & Claiming Childhood Trauma

"There is a time for everything,
and a season for every activity under the heavens."

Ecclesiastes 3:1-8

1. Have you ever had an experience in your life that you would term as traumatic? Yes   No   If so, why?

_____
_____
_____
_____
_____
_____
_____
_____

2. Did you feel loved and lovable in your youth? Yes   No   Please explain:

_____

_____

_____

_____

_____

_____

_____

3. Do you feel loved and lovable now in your adult years? Yes   No   Please explain:

_____

_____

_____

_____

_____

_____

_____

4. What words or phrases would you use to describe your childhood experience?

_____

_____

_____

_____

_____

_____

_____

5. Was there anyone in your childhood that made your life difficult? Please describe:

_____

_____

_____

_____

_____

_____

_____

6. Is there someone in your life now who creates a strain in your life? Please explain:

_____

_____

_____

_____

_____

_____

_____

7. Is there someone in your life who is supportive of you through thick and thin? If so, in what way(s)?

_____

_____

_____

_____

_____

_____

_____

8. Do you have someone you can talk with about whatever is on your mind and heart?

9. How do you relieve stress in your life?

10. When you feel hurt, how do you usually respond? Do you cry, get angry, retreat? Please describe:

_____

_____

_____

_____

_____

_____

_____

11. Repressing emotions can cause physical problems such as headaches, gastric upset, and the like, as well as, mental health issues like depression, anxiety, and post-traumatic stress disorder, or PTSD. When you have strong emotions, are you able to talk them out or do you hold them in hoping they will dissipate and go away? If so, is there another way to handle emotions so they do not get internalized?

_____

_____

_____

_____

_____

_____

_____

12. Have you ever had stress affect your physical health?
    Yes   No   Please describe:

_____

_____

_____

_____

_____

_____

_____

_____

Chapter 5 Questions
Uncharted Waters: The College/Early Adult Years

"So do not fear, I am with you; do not be dismayed,
for I am your God. I will strengthen you and help you;
I will uphold you with my righteous right hand."

Isaiah 41:10

1. Have you ever found yourself in a vulnerable place in uncharted waters? Yes   No   If yes, please describe:

_____
_____
_____
_____
_____
_____
_____

2. How did you know you were in uncharted waters? Please explain:

_____

_____

_____

_____

_____

_____

_____

3. Where do you turn for help when you feel down or vulnerable?

_____

_____

_____

_____

_____

_____

_____

4. Can you think of a difficult time in your life when God helped you reach higher ground?

___

5. Living 'in the day' is a choice we all have to make. Do you find it challenging living in the moment, living one day at a time?

___

6. Have you ever found yourself 'living in the edge?' Please describe:

_____

_____

_____

_____

_____

_____

_____

7. If you have a time when you were 'living on the edge,' what changed for you to get you to higher ground?

_____

_____

_____

_____

_____

_____

_____

8. Were you able to pray and ask for God's help? Yes   No   What was the outcome?

_____

_____

_____

_____

_____

_____

_____

Chapter 6 Questions
Settling Down

*"This is the day which the LORD has made.
Let us rejoice and be glad in it."*

Psalm 118:24

1. How would you describe your life from 19 to 22 years of age?

_____

_____

_____

_____

_____

_____

_____

_____

2. Was that age a turbulent time for you? If so, why?

_____

_____

_____

_____

_____

_____

_____

3. Have you ever experienced a traumatic experience in your youth? Adulthood? If so, please describe:

_____

_____

_____

_____

_____

_____

_____

4. What is the source of your greatest fear?

_____

_____

_____

_____

_____

_____

_____

5. What is your greatest strength?

_____

_____

_____

_____

_____

_____

_____

6. Everyone has strengths and weaknesses; what is an area you would like to work on in your life?

_____

_____

_____

_____

_____

_____

_____

7. Do you have a major accomplishment that you have met in your life? If so, what?

_____

_____

_____

_____

_____

_____

_____

8. List 5 goals you have for your life:

_____

_____

_____

_____

_____

_____

_____

9. List 3 goals you have accomplished in your life:

_____

_____

_____

_____

_____

_____

10. Is there anything that has detoured you from achieving your goals?

_____

_____

_____

_____

_____

_____

_____

11. Have you ever had a time in your life that felt like an emotional roller coaster? Describe:

_____

_____

_____

_____

_____

_____

_____

12. Are you aware of a special time in your life when God has blest you?

_____

_____

_____

_____

_____

_____

_____

_____

Chapter 7 Questions
Untreated Childhood Trauma:
Fertile Ground for Depression, Autoimmune and Neurological Illnesses

"Come to me, all you who are weary and burdened, and I will give you rest."

Matthew 11:28

1. Medical research has discovered that emotional trauma sometimes enters the body via the immune and neurological systems. Do you personally know anyone who has "the trifecta," including depression, auto-immune disease, and a neurological condition? Yes   No   What are their symptoms?

_____

_____

_____

_____

_____

_____

_____

2. Stress can and does affect our bodies in a myriad of ways. Do you often get colds, headaches or gastric conditions such as upset stomach, irritable bowel syndrome, or IBS, or ulcers that require seeing your doctor? If so, how often per year?

_____

_____

_____

_____

_____

_____

3. Have you ever been diagnosed with an auto-immune or neurological condition of unknown origin? If so, please describe:

_____

_____

_____

_____

_____

_____

4. Do you have a history of depression, in combination with, an auto-immune or neurological condition? If so, please describe:

_____

_____

_____

_____

_____

_____

_____

5. Have you ever been diagnosed with or been hospitalized for clinical depression, depression lasting longer than 3 weeks? Yes   No   If yes, please describe:

_____

_____

_____

_____

_____

_____

_____

6. Have you ever been told that you have PTSD? If so, describe what that entails for you:

_____
_____
_____
_____
_____
_____
_____
_____

7. Have you ever experienced clinical depression? Yes   No   How did you know you weredepressed? Please explain:

_____
_____
_____
_____
_____
_____
_____
_____

8. Research tells us that approximately 20.9 million Americans live with depression. Have you ever felt hopeless, disinterested in things that you normally enjoy or sick with vague symptoms? Yes   No   Describe the symptoms you experienced:

_____

_____

_____

_____

_____

_____

_____

9. Do you have insomnia or trouble staying asleep two or more nights per week? Yes   No   Do you know what keeps you awake?

_____

_____

_____

_____

_____

_____

_____

10. Have you ever been diagnosed with an auto-immune disorder and depression? Yes   No   Please describe your symptoms:

_____

_____

_____

_____

_____

_____

11. Have you ever seen a doctor for panic attacks? Yes   No   What was the experience like?

_____

_____

_____

_____

_____

_____

12. If you have ever been diagnosed with depression or anxiety, did it require anti-depressant medication to treat the problem? Yes   No   Did the medication help you? Please explain:

_____

_____

_____

_____

_____

_____

_____

Chapter 8 Questions
The Mind-Body-Faith Phenomenon©

"They that wait upon the Lord shall renew their strength..."

Isaiah 40:31

1. Have you ever prayed for yourself or someone else for healing? If so how did you pray for them? Please describe:

_____
_____
_____
_____
_____
_____
_____

2. In as much as prayers are always answered by God, what were the results of your heartfelt prayers?

___

3. How were your prayers answered?

___

4. What does the term "No shame, no blame" mean to you in terms of mental health issues?

_____

_____

_____

_____

_____

_____

_____

5. The mind-body connection involves shared chemistry between the brain and the body.

    Describe your own mind-body connection symptoms you have experienced:

_____

_____

_____

_____

_____

_____

_____

6. Sometimes people get caught up in the "Medical merry-go-round' going from one doctor to the next. Have you ever had a time where you sought medical help to no avail, and what was the eventual outcome? Please explain:

_____

_____

_____

_____

_____

_____

_____

7. What did it feel like to seek out medical care from numerous healthcare doctors?

_____

_____

_____

_____

_____

_____

_____

8. Have you ever been misdiagnosed, or undiagnosed, for longer than 3 months? Yes   No

   Were you eventually able to get the help you needed? Please describe:

   _____

   _____

   _____

   _____

   _____

   _____

   _____

9. Faith in God can be very healing in mind and body, the antidote to hopelessness and infirmity for some people. Have you ever prayed and felt more hopeful and healthy?

   _____

   _____

   _____

   _____

   _____

   _____

   _____

10. Optimism and positive thinking are important for good health in body, mind and spirit. Do you have a favorite thing you do to help you to cope or have attitude adjustments during negatively charged, challenging times?

_____

_____

_____

_____

_____

_____

_____

11. When faith is introduced into the mind-body connection, it is called *The Mind-Body- Faith Phenomenon©*, and for many people, hope soars. Have you ever had an experience where you prayed and your health improved?

_____

_____

_____

_____

_____

_____

_____

12. Can you think of a time or times in your life when you experienced healing after prayer?

    Please describe:

    _____

    _____

    _____

    _____

    _____

    _____

    _____

Chapter 9 Questions
Silent No More, Victim No More

*"For I know well the plans I have for you;
plans for your welfare, not for woe..."*

Jeremiah 29:11-13

1. What does the term "No shame, no blame" mean to you and how does it apply to your physical and mental health?

_____

_____

_____

_____

_____

_____

_____

_____

2. If you have ever felt like a victim, what were you able to move from survivor to thriver?

_____

_____

_____

_____

_____

_____

_____

3. How did you feel after conquering fear and hopelessness? Please explain:

_____

_____

_____

_____

_____

_____

_____

4. Do you believe that God has a specific plan for you and your life?

_____
_____
_____
_____
_____
_____
_____
_____

5. Do you have a sense of purpose in your life? If so, what it is it?

_____
_____
_____
_____
_____
_____
_____
_____

6. If so, what do you consider to be your purpose(s) in this life?

_____

_____

_____

_____

_____

_____

_____

7. Jesus condensed the 10 Commandments into 2 mandates. He tells us to love God with all our being; and to love each other. How can you show God your love and others?

_____

_____

_____

_____

_____

_____

_____

8. Do you believe that God is kind and merciful? If yes, please explain:

_____

_____

_____

_____

_____

_____

_____

9. How have you experienced the grace and love of God in your life?

_____

_____

_____

_____

_____

_____

_____

10. Has it changed you having God in your life? Yes   No   If so, how?

_____

_____

_____

_____

_____

_____

_____

11. Do you believe God has a plan for each of us? Yes   No   What kind of plan(s)?

_____

_____

_____

_____

_____

_____

_____

Chapter 10 Questions
Moving From Broken to Blest

"The joy of the Lord is your strength."

Nehemiah 8:10

1. Do we seek God first, or does He seek us out first?

___

___

___

___

___

___

___

___

2. Do you believe that God stands in wait for you to grasp His outstretched hand, especially in challenging times? If so, please explain:

_____
_____
_____
_____
_____
_____
_____
_____

3. Have you ever had a time when God helped you out of a challenging spot?

   Please explain:

_____
_____
_____
_____
_____
_____
_____
_____

4. It has been said that faith and fear cannot co-exist. Do you agree? Why or why not?

_____

_____

_____

_____

_____

_____

_____

5. The Bible tells us that "The joy of the Lord is your strength." Where does your joy come from?

_____

_____

_____

_____

_____

_____

_____

6. If the joy of the Lord is your strength, how can you make sure that you stay strong?

7. If prayer is the key to peace and joy as the Bible tells us, what can we do to embrace that truth?

8. How can we draw near God throughout the normal course of our day?

9. How can we welcome God into our lives?

10. What are 5 of the benefits of welcoming Jesus into your life?

___

11. Name 3 Bible promises God has given us through Scripture:

___

12. Be not afraid is written throughout the Bible. What are 2 things we can do to reassure ourselves of the presence of God in our lives?

_____

_____

_____

_____

_____

_____

_____

Chapter 11 Questions
Time to Banish Negative Thinking

*"Be strong and take heart,
all you who hope in the Lord."*

Psalm 31:25

1. Do you experience negative thinking often? Please explain:

_____
_____
_____
_____
_____
_____
_____
_____

2. How do you banish negative thoughts when they arise?

_____
_____
_____
_____
_____
_____
_____

3. Have you ever had negative thoughts that kept you awake at night? Please describe:

_____
_____
_____
_____
_____
_____
_____

4. Are you able to 'change the station' in your mind when negative thoughts arise? Please explain:

_____

_____

_____

_____

_____

_____

_____

5. How do negative thoughts affect your relationships and comfort level? Please explain:

_____

_____

_____

_____

_____

_____

_____

6. How do you deal with negative thoughts as they arise?

_____

_____

_____

_____

_____

_____

_____

Chapter 12 Questions
Contentment: I Have All I Need

*"I have learned the secret of being content in any and every situation...
I can do all things through Him who gives me strength."*

Philippians 4:12-13

1. How would you describe yourself, as a negative or a positive person? Why?

_____
_____
_____
_____
_____
_____
_____
_____

2. Is optimism important to you? If so, how?

_____

_____

_____

_____

_____

_____

_____

3. Do you believe that contentment and peace are important traits that you possess? Please describe:

_____

_____

_____

_____

_____

_____

_____

_____

4. What is the reason for your contentment?

_____
_____
_____
_____
_____
_____
_____

5. 5. How do you define contentment?

_____
_____
_____
_____
_____
_____
_____

6. 6.Describe what it means to be content:

_____

_____

_____

_____

_____

_____

_____

Chapter 13 Questions
Gratitude, Peace and Joy

"May the God of hope fill you with all joy and peace as you trust in Him!"

Romans 15:13

1. Where do you place your trust?

___
___
___
___
___
___
___

2. What brings you peace?

3. What brings you joy?

4. What are you grateful for in your life?

5. How does gratitude to God enrich your life?

6. List 5 things that you are grateful for:

_____

_____

_____

_____

_____

_____

_____

Exercise #2 The Healing Workshop: Quiz: Are You an Adult Child of Trauma?

1. Would you describe your childhood as difficult, abusive, or traumatic? [Yes or No]
2. Did either of your parents (or both) live with an untreated mental illness, or an addiction to drugs and/or alcohol? [Yes or No]
3. Were your parents separated or divorced during your childhood? [Yes or No]
4. Do you have frequent bouts of depression and sadness, emotional highs and lows, anger, panic attacks or anxiety? [Yes or No]
5. Do you have nightmares or flashbacks relating to your childhood? [Yes or No]
6. Do you often get colds, rashes, gastric upset, psoriasis, or infections? [Yes or No]
7. Do you battle fatigue or disorganization in your daily life, having difficulty 'keeping up' with your own schedule of daily activities? [Yes or No]
8. Do you have trouble staying with a job for longer than 2 years? [Yes or No]
9. Do you have an addiction to alcohol, drugs, food, or anything else? [Yes or No]
10. Do you feel like your family often blamed you for things that went wrong in the family? [Yes or No]
11. Did anyone in your family call you the family "an odd duck" or similar? [Yes or No]
12. Were you the class clown in your class at school in your youth? [Yes or No]
13. Were you frequently ostracized at home? [Yes or No]
14. Do you have trouble remembering your childhood? [Yes or No]

Score: Tabulate "Yes" answers

- If you answered "Yes" to 8-14 questions, there is a high probability that you experienced severe childhood trauma survivor.
- If you answered "Yes" to between 5 and 7 of the questions, it is likely you have experienced a moderate level of childhood trauma in your youth.
- If you answered "Yes" to between 3 and 4 of the questions, it is possible you may have experienced some sort of traumatic childhood event.

Exercise #3 The Healing Workshop
7 Ways to Quell Negative Thinking

1. **Identify Negative Thoughts As They Occur**

   Whenever you experience negative thoughts, or experiences, name them and claim them as soon as you become aware of them. This will enable you to continue onto the next step in this vital process of dealing swiftly with negative thinking.

2. **Banish Negative Thinking**

   To isolate and banish negative thinking, it is imperative that you change your thought process.

   This is accomplished by figuratively changing the channel on your TV. It is a conscious decision that requires action on your part.

3. **Escort Negative Thoughts Out Promptly**

   Close your eyes and imagine that someone has entered your home that is not welcome. Now imagine yourself walking them to the door, evicting that person, and closing the door of your home behind them. Evicting negative thoughts is very similar to that. You and you alone are in control of what you think and only you have the power to 'change the channel' whenever needed.

4. **Focus on Positive Imagery** (such as a favorite place)

   When negative thoughts press in, close your eyes and choose to focus on something you either really enjoy, like to do, or a place you love to be. Many people go to their favorite beach in their mind when asked to do guided imagery. Or dancing, or skiing, or crafting. The object is to immerse yourself in positive thoughts that make you feel good. This can also help change your mind-body chemistry, by releasing feel good endorphins that help you stay on a positive track.

5. **Surround Yourself With Positive People**

   The company you keep has much to do with how you think and feel. Surrounding oneself with loving, caring, positive people is imperative for a happy, healthy life. In as much as birds of a feather really do flock together, choosing your friends carefully will reap many benefits for you and also for them. Negative people can bring you down and leave you feeling negative and burdened. Conversely, a caring, loyal friend can be a true blessing, especially through times of great challenge and adversity.

6. **Stay Busy**

   They say that busy hands are happy hands, and it is true! Being idle and alone for long periods of time is never a good idea, as *we all need people, structure, purpose, and activity in our lives.*

   Volunteering to help other people, getting involved in your community, learning another language, bicycling, skiing, exercising, pursuing hobbies like writing, crafting, knitting, tapestry making, or scrapbooking are all great ways to maintain a happy, blest life. These activities can keep you healthy, and stay sharp and focused, and moving forward in your life. They also may serve as a distraction for you from worry, fear, and negativity, while promoting a sense of wellbeing.

7. **'Speak Life' into every circumstance and relationship**

   Rather than speaking negatively, we need to avoid speech that lowers our spirits and pushes us into a state of depression and ultimately, even despair. By avoiding negative speech and using positive speech instead, we are then free to confidently 'speak life' and hope into every circumstance as our perspective is seen through the eyes of faith. Medical research has proven that positive people have more fulfilling relationships and enjoy better physical and mental health than those who are negative. Negative speech is a direct route to negativity, and various forms of depression, and should be avoided at all costs. Clearly, the social, physical, mental, emotional and spiritual costs of negative speech are simply too high to pursue, and must be replaced with life-giving speech that promotes health in body, mind and spirit.

Healing Workshop Questions

1. How does negativity affect your overall health and mood?

   _____
   _____
   _____
   _____
   _____
   _____
   _____

2. In general, how does optimism affect your overall health and mood?

   _____
   _____
   _____
   _____
   _____
   _____
   _____

3. We all get to choose what we think about. How do you evict negative thoughts before they can take root?

_____

_____

_____

_____

_____

_____

_____

4. How can you become more optimistic in the face of challenges?

_____

_____

_____

_____

_____

_____

_____

5. Name 3 ways to quell negative thinking and make way for positive thoughts:

___

6. Early identification of negative thoughts is vitally important to positive thinking. How can you raise your own awareness of negative thought patterns?

___

Exercise #4 The Healing Workshop: 7 Steps to Move From Broken to Blest

Though there will be some overlap, each step in this process is vitally important to initiate before the next step. Forgiveness is at the hub of effectively being able to put aside childhood trauma, each section is covered below in more detail:

Step 1: Acknowledge Your Brokenness

Step 2: Invite Jesus to Come Into Your Life

Step 3: Evict Negative Thoughts about Yourself and Others

Step 4: Reach For Forgiveness: The Key to Health and Happiness

Step 5: Accept Your Own Imperfections & Those of Others

Step 6: Learn to Look For Silver Linings in Adversity

Step 7: Embrace the Healing That Awaits You

Workshop Questions:
Moving From Broken to Blest

"The joy of the Lord is your strength."

Nehemiah 8:10

1. Do you have any heartaches, grief, or areas in your life where you experience brokenness?

_____

_____

_____

_____

_____

_____

_____

2. All of us have at times felt broken in some way. Describe a time when you personally experienced brokenness:

_____
_____
_____
_____
_____
_____
_____

3. Were you able to pull out of your brokenness or did you need help from a friend or a professional? Please explain:

_____
_____
_____
_____
_____
_____
_____

4. What does it mean to evict negative thoughts?

___

5. List 3 specific things you have done to move your own life from broken to blest:

___

6. Medical research reveals that optimism is vitally important for good health. What are some ways to boost your own optimism?

_____

_____

_____

_____

_____

_____

_____

7. The anxiety that comes with perfectionism can be daunting for most people. What can you do to accept your own imperfections and those of others, thereby improving your overall well-being?

_____

_____

_____

_____

_____

_____

_____

8. Looking for "silver linings" in adversity is one important way to cope with life as it evolves. How do you find silver linings in your life?

_____

_____

_____

_____

_____

_____

_____

9. Faith is one way to boost optimism as you pray and trust in God to help you. Can you think of a time you prayed and your optimism increased?

_____

_____

_____

_____

_____

_____

_____

10. If not though prayer to God, where does your help come from?

_____

_____

_____

_____

_____

_____

_____

11. According to the Holy Bible, God's love is for all people. Is there anyone you can think of that is beyond God's reach? If so, why?

_____

_____

_____

_____

_____

_____

_____

12. Is there any sin that cannot be forgiven by God, any condition that He cannot heal?

Exercise #5 The Healing Workshop: Memory Lane: How to Start a Healing Journal

> *'He who was seated on the throne said,*
> *"I am making everything new!"*
> *Then he said,*
> *"Write this down, for these words*
> *are trustworthy and true."'*
>
> Rev. 21:5

10 Easy Steps to Getting Started Journaling

1. Use a computer, pad of paper, spiral notebook or journal to write your Healing Journal.
2. Try to find a comfortable regular writing place where you are free from distractions.
3. Decide on a regular time of day to journal
4. Pray for God's guidance and discernment each time before you write
5. Draw your family tree
6. Find a friend to journal and share with
7. If you had a serious trauma, you may want to find a psycho-therapist to work with you.
8. For maximal mind-body health, if you are not doing so already, begin working on your overall wellness by eating healthy foods.
9. Write down every piece of the puzzle that you remember and soon a fuller picture will emerge.
10. Exercise or walk regularly; walking with a friend is a good way to exercise with regularity to relieve stress and promote good health.

Memory Lane: A Place to Visit, Not to Dwell

Memory Lane. For many people, Memory Lane is a refreshing walk in the park. Yet, for those who have experienced untreated trauma or other difficult life experiences, it is anything but a peaceful jaunt on a sunny day. In fact, for those with untreated childhood trauma, it can be more of a haunting with old tapes running through their mind depicting past oppression, and negative life experiences such as child abuse, neglect, abject poverty, abandonment, rejection, and the like. For people who have had such difficult life experiences, Memory Lane can be extremely anxiety and depression provoking, two feelings preferably avoided at all costs.

For wherever torment rules, there is no peace, and mayhem, chaos and confusion are the order of the day. In essence, it is important to find a way to remove the thorns and shrapnel that permeated your heart and mind, clearing the way for forgiveness, reconciliation, and healing.

This freedom allows you to envision, process and live life to the fullest in new and unprecedented ways. It enables you to look at others with more compassion; to embrace new opportunities with gusto, free of unnecessary internal obstacles, and anxiety, and with minimal fear of the unknown.

Walking in this contentment and peace, you are free to *respond to situations as the needs arise, rather than to react* with almost a knee jerk reaction, able to stay calm in times of challenge, and to be more prepared for fighting off temptations of depression, fear and anxiety.

By so doing you become more able to respond effectively to life as it unfolds on its terms, without everything feeling like a crisis. This new way of responding to situations and peoplecan lend itself to a new way of seeing the world at-large, and to positive behavioral changes that may make a big difference in one's mood, perspective, body chemistry and response to stressful events and circumstances.

Walking in contentment, peace and joy, there is no longer any reason to wait for the other shoe to drop, so to speak. Old thoughts of failure and negative feelings of self-fulfilling prophecy are now met with new confidence and a future full of hope to share. Instead, you can see yourself embracing a sort of truce with destructive negativity, and are more able than ever to live in, and press on, in the present, counting my blessings, welcoming opportunities for growth, and walking in the light of God's peace. Looking ahead with great optimism, you can move forward in any situation, any environment, looking for the best in yourself and others, and, by the grace of God, are able to find it with ease.

There are many benefits to writing out trapped or recurring, traumatic memories as they bubble up in thoughts, dreams, night mares, and even flash backs. First, by writing, you may be able to 'get the negativity out' of your mind, and into the open so you can could better deal with iteffectively. When traumatic memories are kept inside, they often can promote physical, mental, emotional and/or spiritual issues and illness, by fueling depression and anxiety.

Getting these uncomfortable, difficult memories out of your system and committing them to paper is a great way to access and review memories that may be negatively affecting you, paving the way for relief from lingering, anxious thoughts, and deep sadness. These feelings, if left untended, can easily bog you down and affect my mind-body-spirit health, in one fell swoop, leaving you, at the very least, vulnerable.

Secondly, writing a personal healing journal will help provide you with significant relief from the haunting, devastating effects that 'old tapes' can have on the mind, body and spirit.

This can be done with or without a therapist, but the support of a therapist, especially for those who have experienced deep rooted, extensive trauma or those who want maximal healing from journaling untreated trauma. A good therapist can also provide much needed emotional comfort and support as difficult memories bubble up.

Thirdly, when you are able to access memories as they bubble up and make themselves known to you, you can start writing in your healing journal using it as a sort of depository for traumatic memories. Journaling is a wonderful way to get clarification and validation for yourself, to reframe difficult memories, make sense of, and peace with, wherever you have been in the past, while removing whatever hurts have embedded themselves in your heart and mind. Journaling, combined with therapy, can help you gain much needed insight into yourself and your life in the here and now. Though the *past is a place to visit, not to dwell.*

Some memories come to mind spontaneously, others in dreams and nightmares while asleep, while yet others come in PTSD flashbacks while awake during the day. Initially, you may not know what to do with all the flooding memories. But it may simply signal that it is time to deal with your traumatic memories so you can begin to heal, let them go, and more effectively live your life with peace of mind.

At first, you may not know what to do with distressing memories, but if you begin writing them all down, you may get some clarity. Consulting a psychotherapist and psychiatrist who is capable and supportive may be most helpful—even necessary for some people. The result may be that, over time, the flashbacks and/or nightmares may slowly subside. Initially, you may see no relief.

However, soon you may experience more satisfying relationships, better sleep, more energy during the day, better physical health even begin to improve your overall wellness.

You may begin to grow in compassion for yourself and those who have hurt you, recognizing their humanness, and your own, like never before. Best of all, the journaling process also allows you to pray specifically, and with clarity, for those who had hurt you most. Yes, healing has a way of bringing us to our knees in prayer. Like discovering pieces of a puzzle, or a mosaic, you can diligently write down what comes to you one memory at a time.

Through journaling, you may also come to recognize the etiology of your own brokenness, and to grow in lasting compassion for your hurting inner child. The extent of accepting your humanness and subsequent brokenness, may even seem to reach beyond your own emotional pain.

Some people find that journaling is best accomplished with the help and support of a good, supportive psychotherapist to guide them. Like a tour guide on a safari, a good psychotherapist can lead you into uncharted waters and onto unexplored land with ease. The overall effect is sort of like going through a dental extraction for an abscessed tooth with Novocain as opposed to without it. Either way, the tooth needs to come out or you risk having the infection affect your overall health. However, it is a choice as to whether or not you use analgesia, or in the case at hand. You get to choose if you want to have an experienced psychotherapist to act as a guide and buffer for the realities that you must face to heal.

In truth, for some people, 'going down Memory Lane' can be a painful experience, as well as, a beneficial life-changing adventure. Having a compassionate, capable psychotherapist onboard to help is a bonus as he or she can often help to soften the emotional impact and guide you through the process more quickly than if you 'go it alone.' Either way, the goal is to take baby steps and wade through the untreated trauma so you can get on with your life, relationships, career, etc... and find peace, joy and happiness in your world. Whether consciously aware of it or unconsciously affected by it, untreated trauma has a way of stopping a person in their tracks.

Infirmity, disability, and emotional torment are all possible, likely effects of retaining or stuffing experiences such as untreated trauma, abuse and/or neglect. You have suffered long enough with trying to be stoic and avoiding the pain of such early life experiences. Maybe it is time for you to step up to the plate and deal with your own grief and innocence lost; time to put aside your fears and trembling and embrace your own inner healing. Maybe your time has come... Perhaps your quality of life, relationships, success, and happiness all depend on healing those old wounds.

The Healing Journal Workshop

1. How would you describe the trauma you experienced? *Circle one of the following:*

   An event   Ongoing   Frequent   A series of events

2. Circle any of the following that you have experienced in your childhood:

   Physical Abuse

   Mental Abuse

   Emotional Abuse

   Spiritual Abuse

   Depression

   Anxiety

   Frequent or Ongoing Physical Illness/Trauma

   Social isolation

   Neglect

   Abandonment

   Rejection

   Shame

   Poverty

   Other: _____

3. Describe your childhood and any abuse or neglect that you are aware of that may have occurred:

_____
_____
_____
_____
_____
_____
_____
_____

4. Were you able to tell a parent, a teacher, the school nurse or any adult that you trusted about what happened to you as a child? If not, why not?

_____
_____
_____
_____
_____
_____
_____
_____

5. Did your parent(s) believe you when you shared what happened?
   Yes   No

___

6. Forgiveness is a gift you give yourself. Is there anyone you feel that you need to forgive relating to your childhood / trauma?
   Yes   No   Please explain:

___

7. If yes, do one of the following activities:

    Write their name(s) on a chalk board or dry erase board. Say aloud: *"In the name of Jesus, I forgive* _____
    Now, erase their names after on the chalk board or dry erase.

    Write their name(s) in the sand at the beach then watch the ocean water wash over and remove their names symbolizing forgiveness.

    Write their name(s) in the snow, then erase it by making a snowball and throwing it.

8. How did writing their names and erasing them make you feel? Please describe

    _____
    _____
    _____
    _____
    _____
    _____
    _____
    _____

9. Write a short prayer thanking God for what you have learned through your traumatic childhood experience: Were there any caring adults or counselors that helped validate your experience with you? If so, who? Please describe:

_____
_____
_____
_____
_____
_____
_____

10. Was there anyone who tried to help you that you need to thank relating to your early trauma? If so, why? Please explain:

_____
_____
_____
_____
_____
_____
_____

11. Was there any possible good, or a silver lining, that came from your childhood?

___

12. The Bible tells us we should always be ready to give the reason for our hope. what is the reason for your hope now, and why?

___

13. Would you recommend journaling to a friend? Why or why not?

_____

_____

_____

_____

_____

_____

_____

14. If God is the reason for your hope now, and you see any blessings that came from your journaling about your childhood / trauma, please describe:

_____

_____

_____

_____

_____

_____

_____

*"Do not fear, for I am with you;
Do not be dismayed, for I am your God.
I will strengthen you and help you;
I will uphold you with my righteous right hand."*

Isaiah 41:10 (NIV)

If this book has touched you in any way, and you would like to contact Adele M. Gill, please send email to: frombrokentoblest@gmail.com

References

1. New International Version Bible, (NIV)

2. New American Bible, World Catholic Press, 1991

3. 'The Numbers Count: Mental Disorders in America,' National Institutes of Health publication,

4. PTSD: A Growing Epidemic, NIH Medline Plus Magazine (online), Winter 2009 issue: Volume 4, Number 1, pages 10-14

5. 'The Purpose Driven Life,' Pastor Rick Warren, author, 'Optimism and Health: A Meta-Analytic Review,' Annals of Behavioral Medicine, June 2009; 37(3) pp.239-256, Heather N. Rasmussan, Michael F. Scheier, B. Greenhouse

6. 'Positive Thinking: Stop Negative Self-Talk to Reduce Stress,' Mayo Clinic, online

7. 'Optimum Health Benefits, Looking on the Bright Side,' The Journal of Personality

8. 'Study: Optimistic Patients Have Higher Levels of Good Cholesterol,' Harvard School of Public Health, 2013

9. 'Optimistic War Vets Had Lower Rate of Depression and PTSD,' Dr. Dennis Charney

10. 'Severe Depression Linked With Inflammation in the Brain,' Medical News Today, Jan. 29th, 2015, David McNamee. Centre for Addiction and Mental Health's (CAMH) Campbell Family Mental Health Research Institute

11. 'Religion, Spirituality, and Health: The Research and Clinical Implications' ISRN Psychiatry. 2012; 2012: 278730. Published online 2012 Dec 16. Harold G. Koenig

12. Modes of Hoping: Understanding hope and expectation in the context of a clinical trial of complementary and alternative medicine for chronic pain, Emery R Eaves, Cheryl Ritenbaugh, Mark Nichter, Allison L. Hopkins, Karen J Sherman, Explore (NY) Author manuscript; Published in final edited form as: Explore (NY). 2014 Jul-Aug; 10(4): 225–232. Published online 2014 April 19.

13. 'How Strong is the Link Between Inflammation and Depression?' Cleveland Clinic News Wire, March 19th, 2015, Brain & Spine Team

14. 'Optimism and Your Health,' Harvard Health Publications, Harvard Medical School, http://www.health.harvard.edu/heart-health/optimism-and-your-health

15. Religious versus Conventional Psychotherapy for Major Depression in Patients with Chronic Medical Illness: Rationale, Methods, and Preliminary Results, *Harold G. Koenig,* Depress Res Treat. 2012. Published online 2012 June 13.

Resource Books

1. The New American Bible, Most Reverend Daniel E Pilarczyk, 1991 World Book Publishers, Canada (NAB)

2. New International Version Bible (NIV), Bible Gateway(online)

3. Patient Persistence, Gill, Adele M., 2000, EP Press, Oradell, New Jersey

4. 7 Pathways to Hope, Gill, Adele M., 2011, American Book Publishing, Salt Lake City, UT

5. Children of Trauma, Middleton-Moz, Jane, 1989, Health Communications, Inc., Deerfield Beach, FL

6. Daddy Where Were You?, Harpham, Heather, 1984, Aglow Publications, Lynnwood, WA

7. Jesus Calling, daily devotional, Sarah Young

8. <u>Religiously Integrated Cognitive Behavioral Therapy: A New Method of Treatment for Major Depression in Patients With Chronic Medical Illness</u>. Michelle J. Pearce, Harold G. Koenig, Clive J. Robins, Bruce Nelson, Sally F. Shaw, Harvey J. Cohen, Michael B. King. Psychotherapy (Chic) Author manuscript; available in PMC 2015 June 5. Published in final edited form as: Psychotherapy (Chic). 2015 March; 52(1): 56–66. Published online 2014 November 3

9. Spirituality and Health, Arndt Büssing, Klaus Baumann, Niels Christian Hvidt, *Harold G. Koenig*, Christina M. Puchalski, John Swinton, Evidence Based Complementary Alt. Med. 2014. Published online 2014 January 30.

10. Religious and Spiritual Factors in Depression, Sasan Vasegh, David H. Rosmarin, *Harold G. Koenig,* Rachel E. Dew, Raphael M. Bonelli. Depress Res Treat. 2012. Published online 2012 September 18.

11. Religion, Spirituality, and Health: The Research and Clinical Implications. *Harold G. Koenig.* ISRN Psychiatry. 2012. Published online 2012 December

12. You Are My Beloved. Really?, *Harold G. Koenig*

Prayers

1. **Divine Mercy Prayer**

   Oh my Jesus, forgive us our sins, save us from the fires of hell, and *lead all souls to Heaven, especially those in most need of your mercy. Amen!*

2. **The Our Father: The Forgiveness Prayer**

   Our Father who art in Heaven, hallowed be thy name. Thy Kingdom come, Thy will be done, on earth as it is in Heaven. Give us this day our daily bread, and forgive us our trespasses as we forgive those who trespass against us, and lead us not into temptation, but deliver us from evil. Amen

3. **The Apostle's Creed**

   I believe in God, the Father Almighty, Creator of heaven and earth.

   I believe in Jesus Christ, his only Son, our Lord, who was conceived by the Holy Spirit, born of the Virgin Mary, suffered under Pontius Pilate, was crucified, died, and was buried; he descended to the dead. On the third day he rose again; he ascended into heaven, is seated at the right hand of the Father, and will come again to judge the living and the dead.

   I believe in the Holy Spirit, the holy catholic church, the communion of saints, the forgiveness of sins, the resurrection of the body, and the life everlasting. Amen!

4. **Prayer of St Francis**

   "Lord, make me an instrument of your peace...Where there is hatred, let me sow love;

   Where there is injury, pardon; where there is discord, union. Where there is doubt, faith;

Where there is despair, hope; where there is darkness light; Where there is sadness, joy.

Grant that we may not so much seek to be consoled as to console; to be understood as to understand; To be loved, as to love.";

"For it is in giving that we receive; it is in pardoning that we are pardoned;

And it is in dying that we are born to Eternal Life."

5. The Beatitudes/Sermon on the Mount

Blessed are the meek, for they will inherit the land.

Blessed are they who hunger and thirst for righteousness, for they will be satisfied.

Blessed are the merciful, for they will be shown mercy.

Blessed are the clean of heart, for they will see God.

Blessed are the peacemakers, for they will be called children of God.

Blessed are they who are persecuted for the sake of righteousness, for theirs is the kingdom of Heaven.

Blessed are you when they insult you and persecute you and utter every kind of evil against you falsely because of me. Rejoice and be glad, for your reward will be great in Heaven. Thus they persecuted the prophets before you."

Matthew 5:3-12 / NIV

CPSIA information can be obtained
at www.ICGtesting.com
Printed in the USA
FSOW02n1237061117
40836FS